TRANSFORMING STRESS INTO POWER

THE ENERGY DIRECTOR SYSTEM

Mark J. Tager, M.D.
Stephen Willard

To our wives, Carol and Merce, and our kids, who shared so much love and support with us.

To our friends, who contributed their unique energy techniques, and

To our many seminar participants, who helped shape the content and skills in this book.

Published by Great Performance Inc.
14964 NW Greenbrier Parkway
Beaverton, OR 97006
Phone 503/690-9181
800-433-3803

Manufactured in the United States of America

Table of Contents

Introducing the Energy Director System

Toward a New Understanding

First of all, let's dispel one big myth about one of the most intimidating and misunderstood words in our language—**stress**. When we hear this word, most of us think of it as an evil that will somehow invade our lives and cause high blood pressure, strokes, ulcers, and other serious maladies. We fear stress as an uncontrollable enemy, and feel we are at its mercy.

The truth is that our *misconception* of stress is the real enemy, not the stress itself. Stress is not an affliction or a disease. Stress is only a force—a very powerful one that involves awareness, attention, and *energy*. But stress is not uncontrollable; you have the choice of using its force to your advantage, or letting it take advantage of you.

If you choose to channel stress, it can empower you. If you let stress control you, your resulting *distress* will certainly be harmful to your body, your mind, and your spirit.

Stress and Empowerment

If we were to ask you, right now, to list the positive ways in which you manage stress, chances are you'd be able to easily identify a handful of tips. "Take a walk, talk with a friend, read a spy novel, exercise, listen to calming music, play with the kids"—these are just a few common stress relievers.

Most of us have a few techniques for handling stress that we rely on *if* we remember to use them; unfortunately, because we're comfortable with them, we often continue to rely on them even when they're not effective in every situation. For example, perhaps you have been able to "burn off" the tensions of work in the past with an exercise program. But as the demands of the job increase, you may find that physical activity alone is no longer enough to meet your stress. What will help us, then, to handle the demands of our increasingly complicated lives?

We don't need to be told that our problems are "all in our head," and that changing our attitude will solve the problem. What we *do* need is to learn how to turn stress into a positive force, both at home and at work.

Work: Meeting Rising Expectations

To beat competition and meet increased work loads, most organizations today are demanding greater productivity from their employees. Employees want and need more resources with which to meet the stress of these expectations. In response, business and industry, government, education and non-profit organizations, hold stress management seminars each day to "quiet the troops." But a band-aid approach to stress management won't work.

How can we help people to recognize stress and harness it effectively *at that moment*, rather than realizing only *after* a stressful time what they *could* and *should* have done? How can we keep people psychologically fit in stressful environments? How can we maximize individual and group energy to meet greater challenges? How can we transform stress into power? We believe that people can learn to successfully channel increasing amounts of pressure, and even thrive on it!

Learning to Handle More

In the pages ahead, you will find a complete system for turning the challenges of stress into power. We call it the Energy Director System because it takes a pro-active approach to stress. When you harness the energy of stress, you use it to control your life. You will no longer be a victim of stress, a *stress carrier*, you will be an *Energy Director*. You will have power.

What's Ahead

How you use this power is up to you. You set the course. You decide the ways to best utilize your power—for personal or organizational productivity, for greater happiness or quality of life. That's what makes this book unique: it recognizes *your* uniqueness and it will help you find your strong points...as well as your Achilles' heel.

In Chapter 1, we'll define stress. We will also focus on the stress/productivity connection and take a look at why some people handle stress better than others. We'll introduce the Energy Director principles.

In Chapter 2, you'll see where stress comes from and why it requires energy. You'll learn how to get more energy by increasing your sources, decreasing your drains, and spending your energy wisely.

Chapter 3 shows you how our system differs from most other programs. Our emphasis is not only on getting more energy, but using the *right kind* of energy for the problems and opportunities in your life. We'll discuss the four kinds of energy in detail. Your energies are uniquely inherent in you, but you can learn to strengthen and direct these energies to where you need them.

In Chapter 4, we'll help you examine what you do with your energy, where and how you direct it, and the different ways you can consciously choose to focus your attention and power.

Chapters 5-8 help you build your skills in the four energy areas, learning for example, in the relationship chapter, how to "move people closer in to the real you," or, in the logic energy chapter, how to improve your decision making. We'll help you to increase your creativity as well as to improve your ability to function in the here and now with grounding energy.

Finally, in Chapters 9 and 10, you'll learn to use your newfound energy in the two environments where most people need assistance—at work and at home.

Let's get started on your own energy-direction skills right now. Because when you're an *Energy Director*, you're in charge!

Transforming Stress into Power

HOW GOOD
AN ENERGY
DIRECTOR
ARE YOU?

1

How Good an Energy Director Are You?

Beyond Stress Management

For many people, today's world offers more than ever before: more choices, more challenges, more demands, more changes. We can do things and go places that our parents and grandparents never dreamed of.

But we often pay a high price for these opportunities, and the price is paid in *stress*. Stress seems to be almost universal these days. How often in the past week or so have you heard (or made) one of these comments?

"The stress of this job is killing me."

"I need to get rid of all this stress!"

"The doctor said my condition is caused by stress."

"If I could only get rid of stress, my life would be perfect."

Hundreds of self-help books and thousands of seminars have sprung up, promising to help you eliminate stress from your life. Wouldn't that be wonderful? We don't think so.

We believe that without stress, there would be no challenge, no growth, no problems to solve, no new worlds to conquer. In short, life would be boring and stagnant.

In the pages ahead we will approach stress as a potentially *positive* force, one that you can control. But first, let's look at its evolution and at what we know about it.

Stress: A Word With Many Meanings

Stress means different things to different people. Psychologists, scientists, and the masses have defined stress in a number of different ways, and we can learn from each definition. A classic definition of stress is *our response to change*. From this definition we see an inevitability: everything is changing from year to year, from day to day, from minute to minute—in the universe, in the world, in our lives, in everyday situations.

This definition shows us a basic conflict: we can group, build, and try to create an order and a *structure* to control our environment, but there are still many events and factors we cannot control. This is brought home almost daily by upheavals of nature (or, in insurance language, "Acts of God"), by senseless random killings we read about in the newspaper, or by the very little but aggravating hassles of life that occur when we have done everything we can and are foiled by the whim of circumstance.

Stress is a natural, normal part of life; in and of itself, stress is neither good nor bad. Stress results from the changes in our lives—those that we initiate, and those that are thrust upon us in the form of demands from others. Some changes we label as "positive" or "good." For example, a promotion, moving, or marriage are all good changes; we are pleased by them. Others we call "negative" or "bad"; these are unpleasing changes that are not intended or desired. Regardless of whether changes are good or bad, they all cause stress and they all require energy.

More Than Just "Coping"

Another, and possibly the most common, definition is that stress occurs when the *demands made upon a person are greater than the resources*. From this definition, a term has emerged that became popular in the mid-seventies and early eighties: "coping." The term suggests that somehow you can do the right things to decrease the demands that are thrust upon you; if you manipulate, you'll be able to get by.

Coping is an extremely helpful concept when people are overwhelmed by tragedy, such as a death in the family or an injury, or are otherwise in the stages of great emotional grief; coping can help those people to hang on until they regain perspective. But coping turns negative when people are permanently caught in it and don't move on through the normal stages of accepting change.

Coping can become a way of looking at and of measuring life. The individuals who become its victims talk of "settling for" whatever they can get, or "just getting by." They are happy just being survivors. Others, who apply energy to their problems, talk about "creating," "thriving," and "taking charge." It's easy to see the difference. Energy Directors give more, get more, and are able to handle more.

Stress and Your Resilience

An engineer building a house or a bridge would have a different concept of stress, and would describe it as *the sheering force or the strain that could be applied to an object without its breaking.* He or she would recognize that each working material in the construction of the house or bridge has a different tensile strength—some are flexible, some are rigid; and that there are some properties of objects that make them special. In planning, the engineer would consider not just the forces applied to the object, but also what makes that object unique.

This uniqueness is at the heart of the Energy Director System; it's helpful to think of yourself as a unique material with your own inherent specifications. By learning to recognize your unique strengths and weaknesses, you'll be better able to anticipate how you'll react to life's pressures.

An Energy Director View of Stress

Our definition of stress is *a force that requires energy.* This force must be met with the right amount and the right kind of energy, focused in the appropriate direction. From this definition come three basic Energy Director principles that, when understood and applied correctly, can make stress work for you.

1. **Energy Directors meet the challenges of life with the right *amount* of energy.** They invest energy wisely by becoming aware of the desires and demands made upon them and how they are responding to those stressors. They pay more attention to issues that are important and can be controlled.

2. **Energy Directors use the right type of energy for each situation.** We have four energies from which we can choose: Grounding Energy, Creative Energy, Logic Energy, and Relationship Energy. Each of the energies has various characteristics, and *all of us have one or two preferred energies on which we consistently rely*. The combination of these four energies make up our unique Energy Profile. People tend to play to their strengths. And since we all have four types of energy—some high, some low—that means that when we continue to call on our strongest type to solve all our problems, life will see to it that we will be wrong 75% (or at least 50%) of the time.

Energy Directors are aware of their unique profiles and recognize their unique strengths. They look for situations that can maximize their special abilities, but they are also flexible.

3. **Energy Directors *focus* their energies to get the best results.** What good is energy if you can't use it to be effective? Effectively channeling your energies includes establishing goals, maintaining your values, and ultimately, attaining balance in your life.

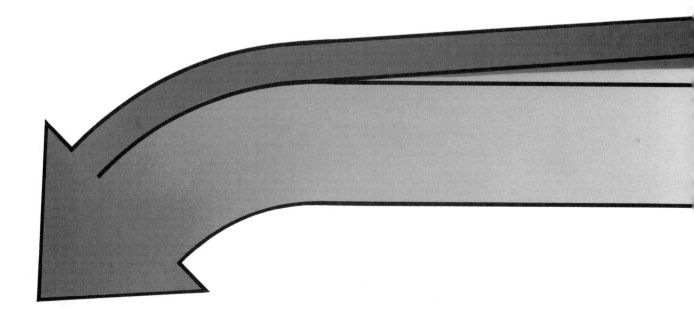

Matching Your Energy

The three Energy Director principles all involve *matching*. We need to match the appropriate amount of energy to meet the demands of the situation, to use the kind of energy that the situation calls for, and to successfully focus our energies on the situation so we can handle it. In the chapters to come, we will learn how to apply the Energy Director principles and match our energies in these three ways.

THE THREE ENERGY DIRECTOR PRINCIPLES

> **ENERGY DIRECTORS:**
> 1. Increase Energy to Meet Stressors.
> 2. Use the Right Type of Energy.
> 3. Focus Their Energy Appropriately.

Throughout this book we will be using these principles to answer a very important question: Why, with two similar people in similar situations, does one thrive on stress while the other breaks? Some people seem to handle stress and use it to make themselves stronger; some are simply and sadly consumed by it. Why? The answer can begin to be found in the stress/productivity connection.

The Stress/Productivity Connection

In the early 1900's, Dr. Robert M. Yerkes and Dr. John D. Dodson, two researchers from Harvard, described a phenomenon that many of us have come to know instinctively: Performance and efficiency are directly related to stress. Their experiments led to the creation of a classic bell-shaped curve, called the Yerkes-Dodson law, that showed how health and performance are affected as stress increases.

To better understand the link, it's easiest to think of the curve as divided into three sections:

Transforming Stress into Power

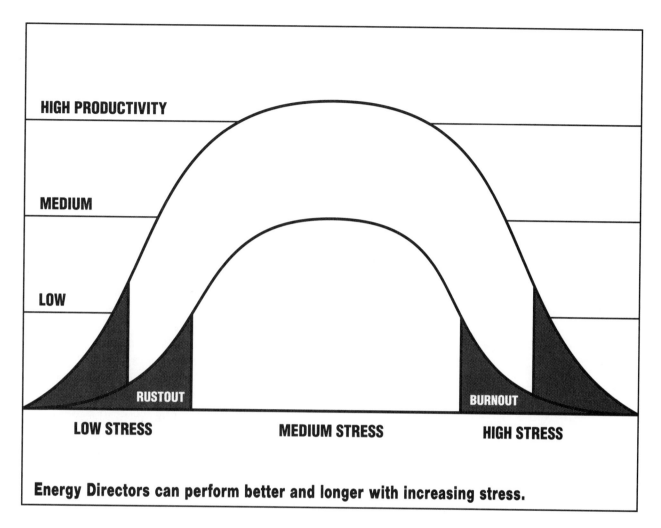

HIGH PRODUCTIVITY

MEDIUM

LOW

RUSTOUT

BURNOUT

LOW STRESS

MEDIUM STRESS

HIGH STRESS

Energy Directors can perform better and longer with increasing stress.

- On the far left end of the curve we have a condition called "rust out." Rust out is caused by a lack of enough stress—enough challenge—to increase drive and motivation.

- The middle of the curve represents an area of solid productivity: moderate amounts of pressure bring forth good results.

- On the far right is a condition commonly called "burnout"—a point at which the body begins to experience the stress response, the warning signs that the effects of tension are beginning to take their toll.

By using the three principles, Energy Directors have learned to extend their performance despite increasing amounts of stress.

Starting on the Road to Energy Direction

Are you ready to direct your energy? Do you want to have more energy, do more with it, and be happier in the process? Before you can even begin, you'll want to examine your attitudes and beliefs about *change*. To what extent do you label changes as challenges, not problems? Do you unknowingly place limitations on yourself that prevent you from experiencing new things in new ways?

Who (or what) is in charge of your life? Studies have shown that people who take responsibility for their own lives are generally healthier, happier, and better able to withstand stress than those who believe they are at the mercy of "fate" or other people.

While we can't control everything in our lives, most of us have a much greater amount of control available to us than we may realize. Energy Directors realize that while they can't always change the stressor, they *can* take control of their response to that stressor.

Many people discover this precise point when they start an exercise program. People who have been inactive often discover that they can do things they never imagined: run marathons, win tennis matches, ski downhill, or climb mountains. This newfound physical achievement spills over into other areas in the healthy forms of greater self-confidence, a new and improved career, and/or better relationships. Their *willingness* to break out of an old routine enables them to see a whole new world.

Are you willing to break out of your comfort zone, to let go of and lose some of the repeating, dysfunctional (those that don't get you anywhere) patterns in your life—to adopt some new behaviors?

Stress and the Repeating Patterns of Our Lives

"I can't believe I did it again."

"I stayed up all night worrying about it, and it turned out to be absolutely nothing."

"If only I had slowed down and looked at the whole situation before jumping in."

"I have a hard time saying no."

Do any of these comments sound familiar? Statements like these reveal that all of us (to one degree or another) are subject to falling into the same old stressful traps. Sometimes we instinctively know the kind of situation that will stress us the most, yet instead of avoiding those situations, we return to them. That's because we are comfortable with our behavior even though it is sometimes unproductive and can even be detrimental.

One of our favorite sayings about embracing change was told to us by an East Indian man: "If you want to make friends with an elephant trainer, be prepared to make room in your house for an elephant." (Or, if you start along a path of change, you may encounter more than you were originally looking for.) Energy Directors have the courage to identify and break through their limitations, so that they can continue to grow.

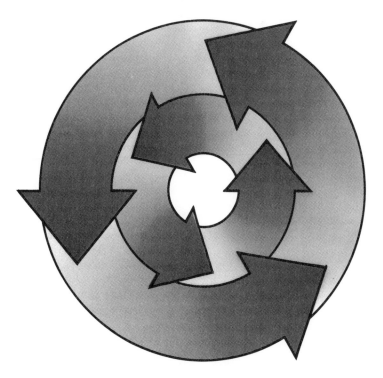

Breakthroughs and the Learning Process

Essentially, there are two components to breaking free from your limitations. The first we call the "AHA!" These are the moments of sudden realization when, in a flash, a problem and its solution are crystal-clear. The other is the nitty-gritty, time-consuming process of learning the skills you'll need to sustain the change. We have a handy formula for the change process. It goes like this:

1. Awareness
2. Knowledge
3. Techniques
4. Practice, Practice, Practice
5. Skills
6. Mastery

First, you become aware of the need for change and gather the necessary information. Next, you learn the techniques for improvement. Then you practice, practice, practice those techniques until you develop a skill. Over time, and through much use of the skill, you achieve mastery. It's the practice, practice, practice part that's the least fun, but it's the activity that gives you the greatest payoff: mastery. Mastery occurs when you are so comfortable using your new skills that you'll use them automatically without even thinking about them. Let's take a moment and assess your energy direction skills.

The Energy Director Quiz

RARELY	SOMETIMES	ALWAYS	*Please answer "Rarely," "Sometimes," or "Always" to the following questions:*
❐	❐	❐	1. Do you identify and monitor your own warning signs of stress overload and do something positive to overcome them?
❐	❐	❐	2. When the demands of work or home increase, can you turn up your energy to meet increased pressure?
❐	❐	❐	3. Are you pleased with the balance in your life between the amount of time and energy you devote to home, work, social, and other activities?
❐	❐	❐	4. Can you easily focus your energy to get things done without being distracted?
❐	❐	❐	5. Are you able to come up with new ideas and innovative solutions to problems?
❐	❐	❐	6. Do you consider others' feelings and anticipate their response when you make decisions that may affect them?
❐	❐	❐	7. When you make major decisions, do you weigh all the factors that pertain to them?
❐	❐	❐	8. Do you take time to gather facts and get enough information to base your judgements upon?

Answers

Questions 1 and 2 deal with your ability to become aware of how you respond to desires and demands, and whether you can turn up your energy to handle increased pressures.

Questions 3 and 4 deal with direction and the concept of focus. It's not enough simply to get more energy; you've got to know how to apply it.

Questions 5-8 cover each of the four different types of energy and your ability to use each kind. If you answered "Always" to all these questions, you may already be a skilled Energy Director. But it's more likely you answered "Sometimes," or "Rarely" to at least some of them.

Energy Direction: A Lifelong Learning Process

By applying the knowledge, techniques, and skills in this book, you'll consistently change those answers to "Always."

Learning is a lifelong process, especially when you're learning about yourself and trying to be your best. No one is a perfect Energy Director (at least we haven't met one yet), but we all have the potential to be closer to this ideal. In reality, life is a trial-and-error process of doing, learning, and refining; of breaking free from old patterns and habits that do not serve you; and gradually, over time, building new ones that can help you achieve your needs, goals, and dreams. In the next chapter, we'll take a closer look at the first energy direction principle—how to match your energy level with the stressors in your life—and we'll cover the skills to help you get started.

DOES YOUR ENERGY LEVEL RISE TO MEET THE OCCASION?

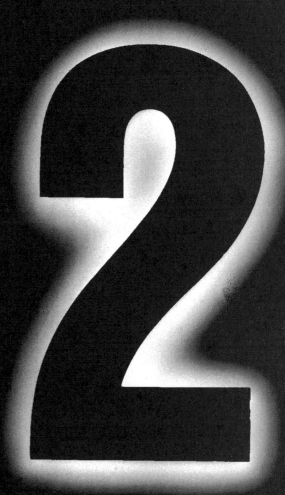

Does Your Energy Level Rise to Meet the Occasion?

It's not such a silly question. We all need energy, of course, but our energy needs differ according to the two categories of stressors in our lives: **desires and demands.**

Desires are *internal* forces. They include our expectations, our wants, our goals, our hopes and dreams. This internal pressure was probably best expressed by the ancient Indian philosopher Buddha, who built a whole religion around the principle that "desire is the root of all suffering." No one today is saying that you have to suffer; but it is clear that, for most of us, when our desires or wants become too great, we experience distress trying to fulfill them.

Demands are *external* forces created by situations or people. Common demands include job responsibilities, family obligations, and life changes. Life changes vary in scope. There are big ones, like moving across the country, and small ones, like moving the living room furniture. Some changes are predictable, such as your kids "fleeing the nest" at a certain age, or your retirement; others, such as an illness or death in the family, are unpredictable.

Desires and demands are often reciprocal, in other words, one causes or affects the other. For example, if you want to advance in your job (desire) you might sign up for additional classes in school. The added burden of classes (demand) stresses you even further. Either way, the more changes thrust upon you, the more energy you need to deal with the situation. Among the most common stressors are:

Expectations: There are three kinds of expectations. In our careers, our personal relationships, our potential in general, *we all have expectations of ourselves*. These expectations are what drive us to perform to our abilities; they're also the basis for self-improvement and growth. *We have expectations of others* (especially children); and *others have expectations of us.* Our parents, spouses, and kids all anticipate that we will act in specific ways. Work-related expectations often take the form of job descriptions, performance reviews, peer pressure, and boss-imposed tasks.

These three expectations, however, are often in conflict. The field of nursing is a classic example. Health care professionals often have high personal expectations that involve compassion and quality of care. They in turn expect their institution to create an environment that allows them to achieve their goals. Finally, patients expect the caregiver to meet their needs. Yet the realities of paper work, political games, and inadequate staffing often prevent caregivers from either fully realizing their self-expectations or meeting those of the patient.

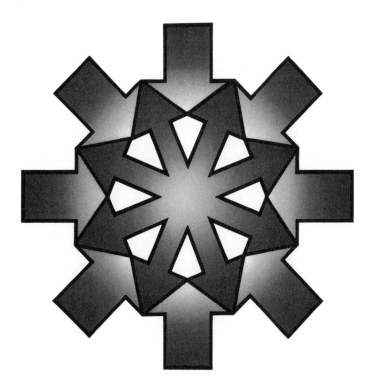

Conflicts with our values: Values are the standards we use to judge our and others' actions. Commonly held values include fairness, trust, respect, and honesty. Sometimes the commitments we form, in acting upon our desires, clash with our values. For example, a fitness-oriented advertising writer may be asked to work on a cigarette account; or an environmentally concerned worker may be employed by a company that pollutes.

Other times, our short-term choices are incongruent—they don't fit in—with our long-term values. If you want to get married and have a family, a long-term value, a possible stressor is a short-term, time-consuming relationship with someone who doesn't want either one.

Commitments and obligations: These are agreements you've made with others—or yourself—that require you to behave in a certain way. Marital fidelity, promptness at work, and your drive to give your employer a full day's work for a full day's pay are all forms of commitment. You may have to sacrifice something in order to remain true to yourself and to those to whom you have made the commitment.

Situations over which we have no control: "There's no use crying over spilt milk" is an antique adage, but it's still perfectly valid today. It's frequently difficult to accept things that can't be changed. Learning to "let go" is an important skill. "Letting go" does not mean you don't care, but merely that you recognize that your added anxiety isn't doing anybody any good.

Time: Demands and desires require time. We can only be in one place and do one thing at a time. Often, when we have multiple demands made upon us in a short period of time, our own personal desires, and our first choices for what we'd like to do with our time, may come last. There is simply no time left in the day to do what we'd like to.

These stressors set off what's called the "stress response" if we perceive them as a threat. If we look at and label desires and demands as problems, we have a crisis on our hands— one that the body responds to in a very predictable way.

Perceived Threats: A Matter of Interpretation

The *stress response* is the body's physical reaction to a perceived threat, and it can be harmful. Until a few hundred years ago, most threats faced by humans were physical ones—an enemy about to attack, for instance. The stress response evolved to help us react quickly to these physical threats. Adrenaline and other chemicals pump into the bloodstream, causing changes like rapid heartbeat, muscle tension, and shallow breathing. Blood diverts from the stomach and intestines and redirects to help the muscles react quickly and strongly. In a few seconds your body has prepared to either fight or flee.

This response is appropriate and lifesaving when we are facing real physical danger—but the fact is, most of the perceived threats we face today are not physical; they're psychological. When your boss is yelling, your kids are making impossible demands, or there's not enough time to do all you'd like to do, your body may react with the stress response. The problem is, that response prepares your body to fight or run away, which won't solve the problem with your boss, your kids, or your responsibilities.

The result is that we often remain in a more or less constant state of distress that upsets our sleep, digestion, and thinking. Long-term tension has been linked to ulcers, heart disease, cancer, and mental illness.

These responses and disorders come to mind when we think of the word *stress*. We think of the stress response—our physiological reaction to perceived threats— and its potentially negative effects on our health.

In general, the stress response manifests itself as one of three forms of *energy disorders*: physical signs and symptoms, thoughts and feelings, and behaviors. The chart on page 22 illustrates some common stress-related reactions.

STRESS? WHAT STRESS?

Umpiring a baseball game certainly looks like a stressful task. Hunched over the plate, pitch after pitch, an umpire must track the trajectory and location of an object traveling up to 100 mile an hour, to determine if it is a ball or a strike.

Three umpires once discussed their philosophy of the job as follows: The first, "It's easy! If it's out of the strike zone, I call it a ball. If it's over the plate, I call it a strike."

The second, "I don't think it's hard. I just call them the way I see them."

The third, "They ain't nothin' till I call 'em."

And so it is with the stressors in life. They "ain't nothin'" until we call them, label them, and give them potential power to affect us.

COMMON STRESS-RELATED REACTIONS		
PHYSICAL SIGNS AND SYMPTOMS	**THOUGHTS AND FEELINGS**	**BEHAVIORS**
Fatigue	Lack of focus	Inability to concentrate
Sleep problems	Nervousness	Overeating
Frequent illness	Irritability	Forgetfulness
Tight neck & shoulders	Impatience	Procrastination
Cold or sweaty hands	Anger	Swearing
Headaches	Low self-esteem	Reckless driving
High blood pressure	Apathy	Oversleeping
Upset stomach	Depression	Drinking and drug use
Fatigue	Helplessness	Negativism
Eyestrain	Hostility	Increase in smoking
Excessive sweating	Loss of confidence	Belittling others
Constipation/Diarrhea	Frustration	Arguing
Nervous tics	Inadequacy	Avoiding confrontation
Rashes	Annoyance	Frequent accidents
Teeth grinding	Anxiety	Hyperactivity

What's important in looking at this list is to realize that these energy disorders (warning signs and symptoms) don't occur in a vacuum. They are responses to the stressors in our lives.

You Begin by Heightening Your Awareness

An Energy Director is more aware of the connection between desires and demands and the ways he or she is responding. How good are you at making the connection between cause and effect? Can you see correlations? Energy Directors bring a sense of heightened awareness to their lives. They use their awareness to monitor signs and symptoms of stress, and use the feedback provided by feelings, thoughts, behaviors, symptoms, and emotions to act. Does this mean that they don't experience distress?

No. They just catch themselves sooner. They make minor adjustments rather than suffer major crises. The length of time from their awareness to their action is shorter.

An Exercise in Awareness

Try the following exercise. Think back to a time in the last few weeks when you were experiencing a great deal of stress. Identify the desire and/or the demand. Now how did you respond? In other words, if a good friend were to observe you, or we could hook you up to a machine that would monitor your body functions, what would we record? Can you link the stressors with your response? Is this one of your recurrent patterns? You might try keeping a log or journal to record events (and your reactions to them). It's easier to see a "cause and effect" when it's written down.

While you can't control all of life's events, you can almost always control your reaction to them. After all, no one else gives you a headache or a stomach ulcer; *you* do it. And acknowledging this control also gives you the power to change.

STRESS LOG	
STRESSOR	**REACTION**

Desires and Demands: Control and Importance

Have you ever found yourself spending ten dollars worth of your energy worrying about a one-dollar problem? How about one dollar of energy on a ten-dollar problem? All of us can identify times when we've done that. *The real goal is to spend energy wisely.* And you'll be most effective when you accurately match up energy and stress.

If you take a moment to think about your desires and demands, you'll recognize that only you can assess their importance, and your level of involvement and attachment to them. What is crucially important to one person may be relatively insignificant to another. You alone determine to what extent you can control or act upon these stressors.

These two factors, control and importance, combine to form a grid with four quadrants, as shown below.

Energy Directors are effective because they expend most of their energy in the first quadrant, the area in which they act upon things that are important and controllable. We've termed this zone the "field of action." They spend little or no energy in the other areas. This conscious choice to spend energy wisely requires awareness, assessment, and appropriate action.

	Important	Not Important
Control	ENERGY DIRECTOR FIELD OF ACTION	
Can't Control		

Let's examine a few situations more closely and see how these principles apply.

Situation 1

	Important	Not Important
Control	Forgot Mother's Day ___ Take Action Call, Send Flowers, etc.	
Can't Control		

You've just realized that because you were wrapped up in a project that required 20-hour days, you totally forgot about Mother's Day. You're actually very close to your parents, care deeply for them, and realize how much you have probably upset and hurt your mother.

You now take time to analyze the situation and label it a +10 (on a scale of ten) in terms of importance. But it is a situation that clearly is within your control in terms of acting to make everything right. You could begin by calling another family member to find out how upset mom was, and then take the appropriate step in terms of calling, sending flowers, a telegram, a gift, etc. The real distress comes when and if you decide to not act, to just accept the situation and assume everything will smooth over in a few weeks.

Situation 2

	Important	Not Important
Control		
Can't Control		Your Pekinese Remark ___ Let Go Don't Waste Energy

You were at a cocktail party with your boss and his wife, who were showing off their prize Pekinese. You made the hasty, off-the-cuff remark, "I've never seen a dog as smart as my cat." You return from the party but can't get the remark out of your head. You mentally berate yourself for the next few hours, wondering how you could have been so stupid. Finally you fall asleep, only to awaken at 4 a.m., again reliving the situation and regretting what you said. The next day you see your boss, who tells you how utterly charming his wife found you, how witty and forthright, and how they'd love to have you over again for dinner.

We have yet to find anyone who hasn't spent a sleepless night needlessly worrying about something that wasn't important (certainly in the big scheme of things), and that they couldn't do anything about. In this example, a little perspective allows you to see the futility of spending energy this way. Hopefully you'll give less attention next time around to such a minor situation.

Learning to Let Go

Other stressors fall into the category of uncontrollable, yet they are important. Being caught in a traffic jam when you're trying to get to an important meeting, having the post office lose an original document critical to the success of a big project, dealing with a terminally ill relative. In these situations, there is much more on the line, yet there is nothing to do but to "let go" of the stressor. Although this course of action seems simple, learning to let go is one of the most difficult of the stress management skills.

To begin with, "letting go" doesn't mean you don't care. You care, but you have learned "detached concern." In this way, the stressor doesn't get to you. Often this ability is only learned with experience, but there are techniques some people use that are helpful. Prayer, meditation, philosophical sayings, and deep-breathing can help to lessen the impact. In some professions, most notably healthcare, this skill is a virtual must.

Reframing: An Acceptance Skill

One of the most helpful acceptance techniques is known as reframing. *Reframing* a situation is a way to look at a "problem" in another light, by creating a new viewpoint that defuses the situation. You can't reframe everything, but you can help yourself with acceptance. To see how powerful a tool this is, consider the following:

It's a cold, rainy night and you have driven around in circles in the parking lot for 20 minutes looking for a place to park. Finally, you notice someone about to pull out and you position your car to take the space, thankful that your ordeal will soon be over. Just as you are about to pull into the space, a pickup truck zooms around you and pulls into "your" parking space. The driver hurries out of the car and runs toward the store, probably trying to avoid a confrontation with you. You tell yourself all sorts of things about how rude and inconsiderate that guy is, then jump out of your car ready to give him more than just a little piece of your mind.

Now let's look at that potentially stressful situation in another light.

The same situation occurs, but this time there are some additional facts. Two minutes ago there was a major accident a half a mile up the road; a number of people were badly injured. The driver of the pick-up truck, having noted the accident, left his passenger at the scene to provide first aid, and was hurrying as fast as possible to the nearest phone to call for life-saving medical assistance.

Same situation, but we'll bet your reaction was totally different—it probably changed from one of anger (maybe even rage) to concern and sacrifice. What has changed has been the way in which you looked at and "framed" the situation. The second interpretation allowed you to reframe it in a way that kept you from defining the demand/desire as a stressor.

Can you find something positive in a problem? Can you suspend judgement? Can you look at an event as a challenge? You can accomplish all three if you put your internal dialog to work.

For people in customer service, having to deal with irate customers is often part of the job. Dealing effectively with these customers is important, but if the situation is beyond your control, there's often nothing much you can do. Yet the heat is still on. At the right is one helpful little device we recommend using when you're under that kind of pressure. Place it in an inconspicuous spot at your work station and repeat the saying to yourself, as needed.

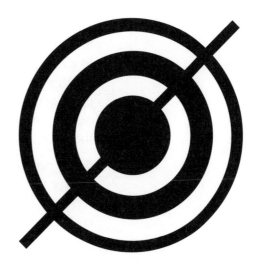

I AM NOT THE TARGET

A Closer Look at Control

Energy Directors do something else that helps them become powerful; they expand their field of action by bringing more and more events under their active control. They challenge the assumption, "There's nothing that can be done." Even when they can't directly transform a situation, they determine whether they can influence it, or if they can predict its effects and respond pro-actively.

Pacing: Racehorses and Turtles

We each have a rhythm or pace that is natural and comfortable for us. Dr. Hans Selye, one of the earliest pioneers in stress research, best summed this up by saying, "There are two types of people: racehorses and turtles. If you're a racehorse, please realize that you have to run. If you're a turtle, make sure to stay out of their way." Remember, though, that turtles are not necessarily less competent or less motivated than racehorses; and racehorses are not necessarily more efficient and capable than turtles. Selye's words merely illustrate the *difference*, and encourage a respect for one by the other.

Racehorse people and turtle people have very different personalities. Racehorses tend to be impulsive and have a greater sense of urgency. They usually speak more rapidly and often finish the sentences of others. They gesture a lot and make quick decisions. They enjoy and are able to handle multiple stimuli coming at them at once, and they like to juggle many responsibilities simultaneously. Turtles prefer to handle one thing at a time and to move more cautiously in making their decisions. They seem calmer and sometimes more focused than racehorses—they don't care much for juggling.

Some people are faster racehorses—and some people are slower turtles. It is a matter of degree that can be represented on a *spectrum* going from *steady* on the one end to *impulsive* on the other.

ENERGY LEVEL

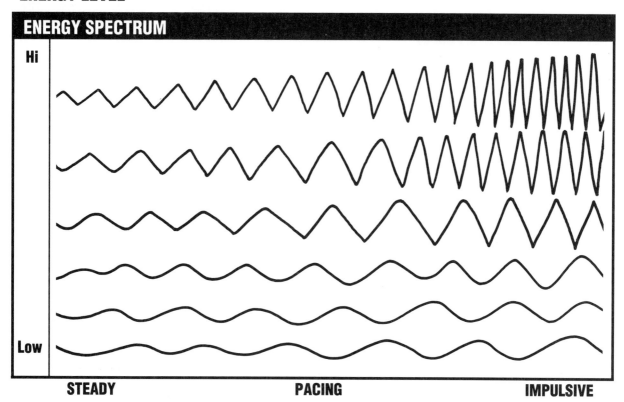

ENERGY SPECTRUM

Hi

Low

STEADY　　　　　PACING　　　　　IMPULSIVE

HOW ENERGETIC ARE YOU?

You can determine your energy level, and measure your pace relative to others, by using the diagram above. On the diagram, draw a box over the area that most accurately describes your energy spectrum. Now place a few other people you know on the diagram. To what extent are they similar or dissimilar to you?

Though each of us has a pace that we are comfortable with, this pace may or may not be what will accomplish our desires or meet our demands. Sometimes we need to use a quick burst of energy to get a project started, even though a slower steady pace is more to our liking. This is an example of a "sprint." If this is not your preferred way to run, you may find that your burst of energy is often followed by a lag or recovery period. An example of a sprint is being told that your boss is out sick and you'll need to give his presentation later in the day. Some people thrive on this pressure. For those who don't, there's a rush of energy, followed by a down period— "I'm too tired to go out tonight."

Other energy demands are called "marathons," because they require larger amounts of energy over time—for example, completing a degree, or working on a long-range project. Here steadiness is the key, and working in impulsive bursts of energy won't get the job done as easily. Both sprints and marathons drive us to perform because of the pressure of both internal and external forces.

Does Your Energy Level Rise to Meet the Occasion?

Increasing Your Energy

In either case, but particularly with marathons, it's extremely important to maximize your *sources* of energy and minimize your *drains*, in order to increase your energy overall. Consider the following:

● Do you know how to get more energy when you need it?

● Does thinking about your goals give you energy? Which goals?

● Do you find that the support and appreciation of another helps you to be more effective?

● Do you use exercise, good nutrition, and relaxation as energy sources?

● When was the last time you "refueled" at an energy source?

Of course, there are no right or wrong answers. What's important is that you be able to identify various sources of energy—and understand how they differ. The energy you get from solitude and meditation, for instance, is obviously far different from the energy you get from a fun party. People, places, things, and emotions are all capable of energizing. Now list the sources of energy that work best for *you*.

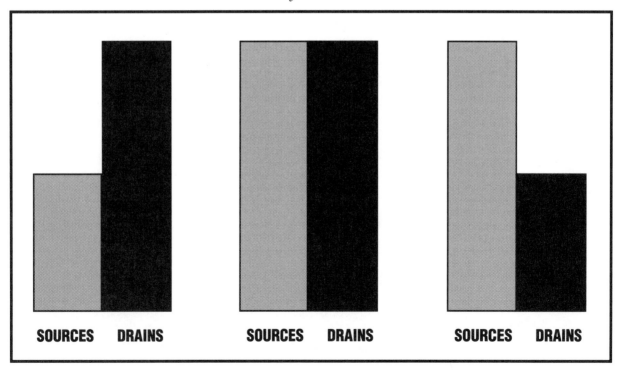

| SOURCES | DRAINS | SOURCES | DRAINS | SOURCES | DRAINS |

Energy Drains

Just as important as where your energy comes from is how you spend it. Do you know where your energy goes? And do you know how you lose or waste it? Getting more energy can often be as simple as plugging up some of your energy *drains*. When we ask people to think of their drains, they often come up with a list that is similar to their energizers. Common drains include:

Other people: There are some people who are "energy vampires." You probably know a few. They are takers, not givers. Most are chronic complainers who always see the dark side of things, and blame others for their problems. They never accept responsibility for their actions. While all of us need the support and encouragement of others, you may wish to re-examine your relationships with these individuals to make certain you're on the receiving end as well.

Your internal dialog: Because only you can determine the amount, effect, and significance of your stressors, the first line of defense is the internal filter that includes our perception of the world around us. This perception is shaped by our *internal dialog*. Imagine for just a moment that we tape recorded your internal dialog for a 24-hour period. What would we hear?

"Stupid. You can't do that. I knew you'd blow it again, Dummy"; or

"Great job. You're doing much better. You can make it happen. Go for it. Now you're on target."

It is as though we have an inner coach constantly monitoring our performance and either criticizing or encouraging us. The first coach creates stress carriers; the second, Energy Directors. Remember that you move toward and become like that which you think about. A healthy internal dialog is a must if you want to transform stress into power.

Poor health habits: These refer to food and exercise. Want to bring your energy level down? It's easy. Every day for a week, overeat by 500-1000 calories, and don't get any exercise. Not only does quantity of food affect us, but quality is important as well. We know that meals high in carbohydrates have, for many of us, a relaxing effect, while those high in protein enhance our mental alertness. And the most valuable kinds of exercise are the ae*robic* ones; they use the large muscles of the body in a sustained way. (More about this in Chapter 5, Grounding Energy.)

Now let's theoretically extend these poor health habits for another month. At this point, a common drain for some people is the excuse that they're "too tired to exercise." They begin confusing the need for sleep with the need for activity, and their energy level can become chronically low.

When you learn to recognize your energy sources and drains, then you can begin to make wiser use of your sources, and diminish or avoid the drains (or face them only when you have enough energy to handle them).

As you develop skills, you will expand your sphere of influence. And as you do so, you will have more power. Energy Directors recognize this. As they grow and become more successful in handling the challenges of life, their sphere of influence increases. They can do more about more things.

By now you realize that stress is a force, one that can lead to illness...or great power. It's time to go forward.

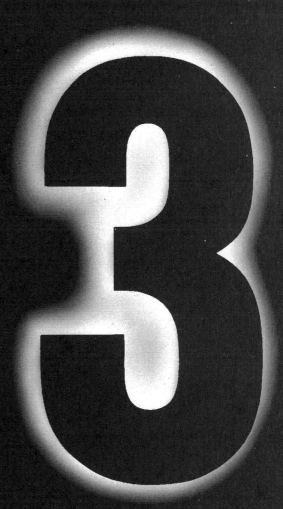

YOUR
UNIQUE
ENERGY
PROFILE

Your Unique
Energy Profile

**Personal Power:
A Complicated Issue**

There's a lot more to being an Energy Director than just getting *more* energy!

If energy were like gasoline, life would be simple. When you're driving a car, a glance at the gas gauge tells you when you're running low on fuel. You find a gas station, fill up the tank, and proceed.

Unfortunately, personal power is more complicated. It's not a matter of just putting in a set amount of fuel to go a certain distance. Not all energies are the same.

There are four different types of energy in our lives:

- creative
- logic
- relationship
- grounding

We all have our dominant energies. Most of us are good at one or two types, and poor at one or two. But it's no use to fall back on our favorite type of energy as the solution to all our problems.

**Energy Differences
Begin Early in Life**

Which energies we favor individually over others is something we learn at a very early age, or even before, because we probably *inherit* tendencies toward one or more types through genetics and hone these talents through interaction with our environment.

34

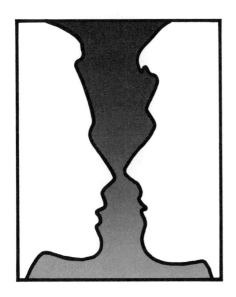

Let's take a closer look at two individuals.

Tom and Jenny are as different as night and day. As a child, Tom was always quiet and reserved. He displayed an early aptitude for reading, and a desire to seek solutions to problems. Not content with simple answers to his "Why?" questions, he always researched topics that interested him.

As he grew older, it became apparent that he liked to analyze situations. He approached problems in a logical, step-by-step manner. Throughout high school he excelled in math and science and always did well in debate. A shy and introverted boy, he didn't mature physically until late in college. Many people first described him as standoffish. Some felt he looked down upon them, thinking that he believed they weren't smart enough to be his friend.

From childhood it was apparent that Jenny was a "people person." The middle child in a family of three, she was always the peacemaker, the one who noticed when her Mom or brothers were upset, or the one who gave hugs and words of support. Jenny was very generous and always shared with the other kids. As she grew older, her popularity mushroomed. She had lots of friends and playmates to whom she often expressed affection. In high school she was elected to class office. It seems that Jenny was always organizing the class events. And, when one of her classmates was ill, she suggested that the class chip in for a present.

Two people with different energy profiles. Let's follow their lives a little longer and learn about their careers.

Tom becomes an attorney for a large Midwestern firm specializing in corporate law. He's respected by his peers and admired by his clients. He seems to be the prototype of the calm, cool, calculating corporate attorney.

Jenny becomes a saleswoman for a computer company. She's well liked by her customers, who are primarily purchasing agents for major corporations in Chicago. She remembers the names of all of her clients, as well as the names of their spouses and children. She knows something about each. Her outwardly friendly demeanor and warm smile make people feel comfortable in her presence.

Why Life Isn't Always so Simple

It appears that both Jenny and Tom have recognized their unique strengths and made the most out of them by positioning themselves in two worlds that let them take advantage of their aptitudes. But, as we'll see in the next scenario, life isn't always so simple and neat. Let's observe an exchange between Jenny and Tom that took place some three months after they'd met and started dating.

Tom has agreed to pick Jenny up at the bus stop on the way to dinner and a play. He arrives, by car, some 35 minutes late. Jenny has been forced to wait outdoors, in the midst of a cold, driving rain, with little protection other than the partially enclosed shelter of the bus kiosk.

"I can't believe you did this to me," she protests. "I've been waiting out here in the cold for more than half an hour. Besides, I was so worried about you I called your office three times, and no one answered. I thought you might have had an accident on the way over."

"What number did you call?" Tom asks, "When did you call? What do you mean, no one answered? You know our switchboard goes down at five. Didn't you have my direct number? You know you should always carry it. Besides, I can't believe you didn't carry an umbrella today. Didn't you listen to the weather report?"

"Do you always have to play the attorney? You know, sometimes I think you just don't have any feelings. Here I am telling you how worried I was and you start acting like the D.A."

"Well, you ought to plan ahead."

"Yeah, and you shouldn't be so thoughtless."

Obviously there's a very real conflict here, but what's behind it? We'll analyze it fully in just a minute, but the important thing to note is that the combatants seem to be sticking to their own type of energy, which they know will work for them in their own environments. **And a mere increase in energy, misdirected, will not solve this problem; it may very well make it worse.**

Transforming Stress into Power

Why are Tom and Jenny having problems? Let's look at their different energies.

Logic Energy

Tom's strength is logic energy. It's the energy of objectivity and analysis. People with logic as their dominant energy are most comfortable dealing with cause-and-effect relationships, not feelings. They relate to the world through concepts and items, create sequences and plans by using existing methods and procedures to solve problems. Highly logical people will often look to the past for data and clues on how to relate in the present and future. They're also more likely to ask *why* questions and await the answers before proceeding with action.

Relationship Energy

This is energy that involves emotions, feelings and concern for others. Jenny demonstrates this energy. People who relate with this form of energy will be highly *sensitive*, both to others and to themselves, and will always be asking, "How will this affect others?" And they have a circular sense of time, often looking backward to compare the present with periods in their lives when they experienced the same feelings. With this energy, there is a tendency toward strong likes and dislikes.

Now let's look at another scenario, involving two other people. Charlie and Barbara are serving on a committee to raise money for a suburban art museum. Like Jenny and Tom, they approach this task from totally different perspectives.

Charlie is a creative director for a large, metropolitan advertising agency. He is one of the most sought-after people in his business because of his seemingly endless ability to come up with ideas. If his clients want one concept, Charlie gives them ten. He is extremely well-read—the type of guy who can participate in a conversation on almost anything. He has the tendency to be a little late to meetings, and is sometimes a trifle disorganized. Some of his co-workers perceive him as being a little "spacey."

Barbara is an auditor for a mid-sized bank located in a remote suburb of the same metropolitan city. She's got all the traits that are ideal for her position: attention to detail and a practical, down-to-earth approach to getting the job done. She demonstrates the same energy in her personal life; her checkbook is balanced to the penny, her world is well-structured—everything has a place. Once she gets on target, she pursues her work with determination. Barbara lives and works in "the here and now."

When Charlie and Barbara come together to work on the art museum fund-raiser, it's like trying to mix oil and water. For Barbara it is an exercise in frustration. Just when it seems that something is about to be decided and a course of action established, Charlie comes up with five new suggestions for the campaign. To Barbara, it seems that Charlie doesn't want to get on with the work at hand.

Charlie feels constrained, feels that Barbara wants to control everything, thinks that Barbara lacks imagination, and that Charlie is not being appreciated for his good ideas.

These two stories, Tom and Jenny, Charlie and Barbara, illustrate one of the greatest sources of stress for people—*conflicts between different energy types.*

Now let's examine why Charlie and Barbara are having problems.

Creative Energy

Charlie demonstrates primarily creative energy. Highly creative people often experience a flash of insight or inspiration that allows them to see situations in a different light, to detect possibilities where before there were only problems. Creative energy is directed toward the future, toward "the big picture" and new approaches. People who feel most comfortable expressing creative energy are usually highly intuitive. They trust their hunches and their first impressions about situations. They tend to work in bursts of energy and remain open and optimistic about life.

Grounding Energy

This is the energy of the "present moment," of the here and now. People like Barbara, who demonstrate a great degree of grounding energy, tend to be practical and oriented toward action. They focus on details and rely on their sensory input to get information about the world. We describe people with high grounding energy as being "down to earth." They are *very* good at noticing details, and base their actions on observations and reality.

The Different Energies: Either/Or

Creative energy and grounding energy are primarily ways in which we gather information. Creative people are in tune with hunches and possibilities. They trust the classic "sixth sense" and can work on very little concrete information. People with dominant grounding energy rely on their five senses to provide them with tangible sensory data about the present moment.

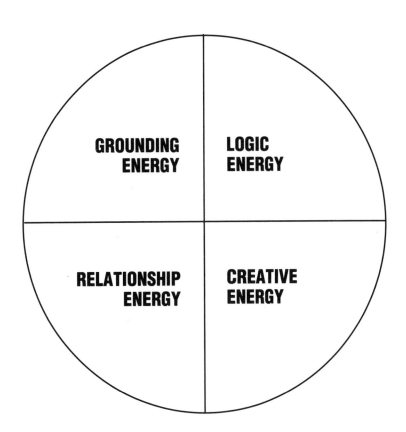

Relationship and logic energy are used to process the information gathered above. People with high relationship energy make their judgments based upon feelings, likes and dislikes, and emotions. With logic energy, decisions are made objectively, based upon facts, formulas, and rational analysis.

The conflicts described in this chapter are classic illustrations of very typical energy mismatches. The people described are being true to themselves and their own experience. Jenny can't understand why Tom is so unfeeling. Tom thinks Jenny is overly emotional and hypersensitive. Barbara has no patience for new ideas, hunches, and impractical suggestions, she just wants to get on with a tangible plan of action. Charlie resents Barbara's desire to limit his creativity.

Energy Directors are Flexible

Each of us has our preferred, dominant energies, usually one or at most two. No one energy is better than others; they are different, and all are necessary in certain situations, and at certain times. We tend to relate to the world with the type of energy we are most comfortable with and that works the best for us. The catch is that one energy type is not always going to be appropriate for all situations. Conflicts often result when people with different energy types take opposite approaches to the same situation.

Energy Directors understand their own energy strengths and weaknesses. They are aware of the effect their energy style has on others. Furthermore, they realize that people are different and they know that to communicate with other energy types, they must be flexible and try harder. All of us can learn to develop our weakest energies through training and skill building... but that doesn't come as easily as using our preferred energies.

Enough of our four characters with their one-dimensional energies. Let's take a closer look at *your* unique Energy Director Profile. Take the quiz beginning on the next page; circle the answer that best describes you. The results may, or may not, surprise you.

ENERGY DIRECTORS: RELATIONSHIP/LOGIC ENERGY

1. When a friend has a problem,

    A. I'm most likely to provide an objective reading of the situation; or

    (B.) I'm most likely to provide emotional support.

2. In making decisions,

    A. I relate choices to my/and others' opinions and feelings; or

    (B.) I prefer being logical, objective, and analytical.

3. Those who know me best would describe me as:

    A. objective, firm-minded, and analytical; or

    (B.) supportive, caring, and empathetic.

4. When I am facing a problem, I would be more likely to:

    (A.) get in touch with my feelings first or talk with a friend about it; or

    B. get a sheet of paper and consider the pros and cons before making a decision.

5. To which statement can you most easily relate?

    A. I hurt others' feelings without knowing it; or

    (B.) I expend emotional energy worrying that I may hurt others' feelings.

6. Which statement describes you best?

    A. I am able to put aside the demands of friends and family to focus on the job at hand; or

    (B.) I have a hard time saying "No" to the requests of my friends and family.

7. Which causes more stress for you?

    (A.) People who won't make a decision based upon the facts that you have carefully presented to them; or

    B. Not living up to others' expectations.

8. In making an important decision are you more likely to

    A. trust your feelings; or

    B. do the logical thing no matter how you feel.

9. Which comes more naturally for you?

    (A.) Expressing feelings; or

    B. Making objective decisions.

10. Which do you feel more comfortable doing?

    A. Sharing vulnerabilities; or

    (B.) Evaluating quantitatively.

11. I like to think of myself as

    A. tough-minded; or

    (B.) tender-hearted.

12. Which comes easier for you?

    (A.) Being empathetic; or

    B. Being objective.

13. Which causes more stress for you?

    (A.) Having to make decisions without enough information; or

    B. Dealing with people who don't consider feelings important.

14. Would you rather be known as a person who is

    A. able to give lots of praise and recognition; or

    (B.) who is fair and just.

15. Which are you more likely to do?

    (A.) Take criticism personally; or

    B. Accept criticism as one input into a situation.

16. Which role is more like you?

    A. Decision maker; or

    (B.) Peace maker.

Look at your answers for questions one to sixteen. Circle the letter you selected for each question on the lists at the right. Count up all the letters you circled in the Logic column and enter the total below. Total the letters circled in the Relationship column and enter that score.

	LOGIC	RELATIONSHIP
1	A	(B)
2	(B)	A
3	A	(B)
4	B	(A)
5	A	(B)
6	A	(B)
7	(A)	B
8	B	(A)
9	B	(A)
10	(B)	A
11	A	(B)
12	B	(A)
13	(A)	B
14	(B)	A
15	B	(A)
16	A	(B)
TOTALS	5	11

ENERGY DIRECTORS: GROUNDING/CREATIVE ENERGY

1. Which describes you best?

    (A.) I prefer standard procedures and proven ways of doing things; or

    B. I prefer to trust my hunches and my ability to quickly come up with solutions.

2. My close friends are more likely to describe me as:

    A. imaginative, creative, and possibility-oriented; or

    (B.) practical, level-headed, and realistic.

3. Which are you more likely to do?

    (A.) Notice details and remember facts; or

    B. Become excited by possibilities and generate alternatives.

4. Which statement describes you best?

    A. I thrive on options, change, and challenges; or

    (B.) I prefer consistency, predictability, and the feeling of stability.

5. Which mistakes are you more likely to make?

    (A.) Failure to anticipate changes, generate alternatives, and seek possibilities; or

    B. Miss obvious facts and details; fail to use standard operating procedures.

6. In a group meeting, which question would you be more likely to ask?

    (A.) What are the facts and what do we do with them?

    B. What are all the possibilities we might explore?

7. To which statement can you better relate?

    (A.) I am more comfortable approaching situations in a tried and true way; or

    B. I am more excited by generating new ideas and moving on to new situations.

8. Which are you better at?

    A. Coming up with ideas, concepts, and visions; or

    (B.) Describing colors, sounds, and physical details.

9. My friends describe me as:

    A. enthusiastic, always changing, and a risk-taker; or

    (B.) stable, predictable, and conservative.

10. Which is more like you?

    A. To keep coming up with another idea; or

    (B.) To be more concerned about how to put an idea into action.

11. Do you:

    (A.) have a good sense of how long it really takes to do a project; or

    B. tend to underestimate how much time projects take to complete?

12. Which would you rather deal with in a job?

    A. Problems that are complex and abstract; or

    (B.) Problems that are clearly defined.

13. What is more appealing to you?

    A. Coming up with your own way of accomplishing something; or

    (B.) Doing something in an accepted way.

14. Which is more difficult for you?

    (A.) Adapting to constant change; or

    B. Dealing with routine matters.

15. Which do you prefer?

    (A.) To live in the here and now; or

    B. To pursue dreams and goals for the future.

16. Are you more likely to work:

    A. in bursts of energy; or

    (B.) with steady, constant energy.

Now look at your answers for questions one to sixteen. Circle the letter you selected for each question on the lists at the right. Count up all the letters you circled in the Grounding column and enter the score below. Total the letters circled in the Creative column and enter that score.

	GROUNDING	CREATIVE
1	(A)	B
2	(B)	A
3	(A)	B
4	(B)	A
5	(A)	B
6	(A)	B
7	(A)	B
8	(B)	A
9	(B)	A
10	(B)	A
11	(A)	B
12	(B)	A
13	(B)	A
14	(A)	B
15	(A)	B
16	(B)	A
TOTALS	16	0

YOUR UNIQUE ENERGY PROFILE

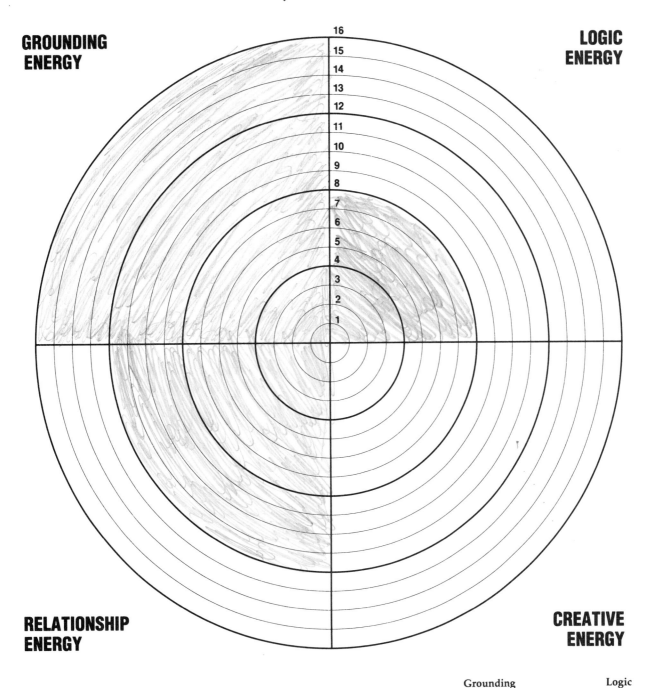

GROUNDING ENERGY

LOGIC ENERGY

RELATIONSHIP ENERGY

CREATIVE ENERGY

Based on the results on page 42 and 44, fill in your Energy Director Profile like the example at the right.

Logic	12
Relationship	4
Grounding	4
Creative	12

5
11
16
0

Grounding Energy

Logic Energy

Relationship Energy

Creative Energy

Stressors and Your Unique Profile

For each of the four energy types, there is also a unique set of stressors common to the people who have this energy. In our workshops and seminars, participants have compiled the following list of stressors. Take a close look not just at the stressors for your energy type, but also for the other types. This will help you appreciate how truly different we all are.

Stressors Affecting Grounding People

Unexpected changes
Last minute situations
Variables that can't be controlled
Having to do several things at once
Indecision
People who change in midstream
People who daydream
Lack of action
Not taking time to plan
Deadlines

Stressors Affecting Logic People

People who don't appreciate facts
People who want things yesterday
Illogical people
Disorganization
Deciding without enough information
Unknown parameters
No focus
Open-ended questions
People who are never satisfied
Having to make quick judgements

Stressors Affecting Relationship People

People who disregard others' feelings
People who don't listen
Rejection and isolation
Taking failure personally
Criticism
Can't say no, overextending oneself
Trying to please others
Guilt
Those who exploit others
"Ends justify the means" people

Stressors Affecting Creative People

Frustration of detail
People who are resistant to change
Having to sit still all day
Rigid rules
Stagnation and the status quo
Procedures and routines
Recycling the same problem
Unproductive meetings
Negative people
Fragmentation

Transforming Stress into Power

Commonly Asked Questions

Is There a "Best" or an "Ideal" Profile?

Absolutely not. Each of us is a unique mixture of preferred energies and acquired skills. Successful Energy Directors have learned to compensate for their weak areas by developing their skills in those areas. In fact, they may compensate so successfully that it becomes very difficult for another person to determine which are their innately dominant energies.

Do People Change Their Energy Profile?

Not without conscious effort. These patterns have been formed and developed since early childhood. Most of us maintain the same energy patterns throughout our lives.

Do Opposites Attract or Do Birds of a Feather Flock Together?

Both are true. Initially we tend to like (or feel comfortable with) people who are most like us in energy profile. It is as if we sense an "aura" about them that makes us feel comfortable. He or she is "just like me". . . "aren't we all wonderful."

We frequently select friends, therefore, who have similar energy profiles. On the other hand, it's not at all unusual to become attracted to or to fall in love with a person with an opposite energy profile. Neither dynamic, by the way, guarantees a successful relationship. (More on this later.)

What if I Have Absolutely None of a Particular Energy?

Relax! It sounds as though someone has labelled you (e.g. "She has no emotions, she's all logic."); you don't have to be pigeon-holed like that unless you want to be. Although some of your energies are stronger and more evident than others, there's an element of all the energies in each of us. Our weaker ones are just waiting to be developed. The Energy Director Profile shows your relative strengths and weaknesses, not the absolute amount of each energy.

Putting All the Energies Together

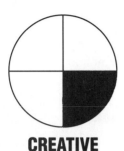

CREATIVE

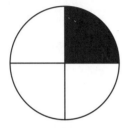

LOGIC

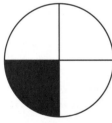

RELATIONSHIP

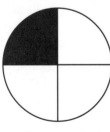

GROUNDING

Remember, the goal is not to balance your four energies; that simply is not possible. What we're aiming at is to maximize your strengths, compensate for and develop your weaknesses, and make the extra effort—no matter how difficult—to deal with situations using the appropriate energy. Life's problems are very complex, and we really need to employ all four energies in some quantity to meet their demands.

Creative energy allows you to see situations in a different light, to detect possibilities where only problems once existed. Using this energy, you begin to grasp solutions and new approaches.

With **logic**, you apply judgement to life's possibilities. You sort and test, analyze and determine. You begin to forge a course, to set a goal and a plan of action.

Most of us don't work alone. Our actions have consequences in the real world. And, for most solutions to be effective, we must make our needs and wants known, while working with and being sensitive to others. This is where **relationship** energy comes in. And depending upon the course of action, we're often forced to deal with the issue of intimacy—how close we are willing to allow people to get to the "real" us.

Finally, **grounding** energy gets the work done. It orients our efforts to the present and the here and now. It involves our senses to gather data which starts the cycle over again, because sensory data is food for the *creative* and *logic* energies.

We will be covering each energy (and how to get more of each) in detail in chapters to come. But first, let's look at the third energy principle, direction.

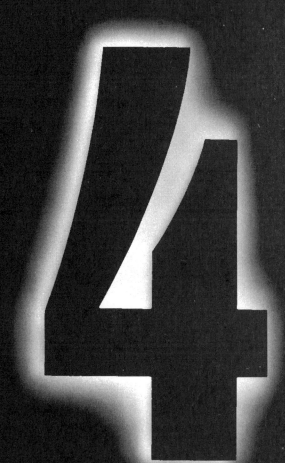

THE
POWER OF
DIRECTION

The Power
of Direction

Our Direction Vocabulary

We can learn a lot about energy direction by listening to the comments people make in everyday life. People talk about their energy being "scattered" or "focused," about being "off-track," or "right on target." There are those days when we are "running in circles" or "spinning our wheels" and others when we are "moving forward" and "making progress." Sometimes we become exhausted by trying to do too many things at once; we feel as though we "lack direction."

There are many aspects to energy *direction*. In this chapter, we are going to simplify them and give you ways to channel your own energy in the direction *you* want. But first, just as there are mismatches with the types of energy, so too are there mismatches in direction that cause stress.

Misdirection and Stress

Imagine for just a moment that you had a few days all to yourself. You could do anything you really wanted during this time. Which would appeal to you more?

A. Three quiet days spent reading a good book, writing a little, playing with ideas and concepts, and having a little social contact with one person at a time.

or

B. A worldwind three days of parties, meetings with other people, and taking part in group activities.

Transforming Stress into Power

Inner- or Outer-Direction

These two situations describe preferences of direction, whether we are more comfortable projecting our energy outward into the world of people, events, and activities, or inward toward thoughts, ideas, and contemplation. This preference has classically been referred to as introversion (inner-directed) or extroversion (outer-directed) and, like the preferred energies, these natural directions seem to be formed early in life.

What appeals to the inner-directed person is exactly what stresses the outer-directed individual, and vice-versa. Here again, we have *potential for mismatches in relationships that involve two people with different natural directions*. We can see this mismatch when an outer-directed and an inner-directed person work together on the same project. Outer-directed people need stimulation. They like to talk to others, "think out loud," and keep moving. Inner-directed people need just the opposite. They want quiet to think through the project or play with ideas. They're more apt to carefully consider what should be done before they rush off to do it.

Short-term Mismatches: The Issue of Focus

The conscious act of focusing awareness is known as "attending." As we've seen, we can attend either to the outer world—events, activities, things, people —or to the inner world of thoughts, feelings, ideas, values, and beliefs. Each person has a natural preference, and this difference can be a source of friction in relationships at home and at work.

Mismatches can occur when we fail to use the right type of attention and direction that a given situation demands. Attention has not only direction but scope to it too; in that respect, it's quite like a camera. We can take in a broad field of view, or we can "zoom in" for a narrow close-up.

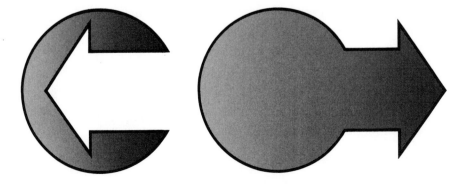

Smarter Space-Planning

Planners of office space would do well to keep in mind that different office environments work best for each energy direction. Many high-tech computer and engineering companies, for example, have "open landscape offices" with shoulder-high dividers between employee work areas. This type of space is fine for employees whose work is highly interactive, but it doesn't make sense for *every* kind of task or worker.

The top managers in charge of planning office space tend to be outer-directed people who thrive on stimulation. Ironically, these executives usually plan closed offices for themselves (the doors of which, they keep stressing, are "always open" to employees), and then put their more inner-directed workers, such as engineers and software developers, in the open spaces. To be blunt, this system is totally backward. It sacrifices interaction on the altar of status, and it forces workers who need to concentrate to work in a noisy environment with constant interruptions. Is it any wonder that those hapless individuals frequently park themselves in closed conference rooms (or in the boss' closed office, when he or she is out of town) in order to get any work done?

We can have mismatches in both direction and scope. On the chart below, we have listed a number of activities that exemplify the different types of focus. Try to picture yourself doing each activity, so you can feel the unique concentration represented by each quadrant.

	Internal	External
Narrow	Adding numbers in your head Mentally weighing pros and cons	Working with tools Using a computer
Broad	Daydreaming Fantasizing	Driving a car Playing quarterback

Now let's examine two typical "snapshots" from life that demonstrate mismatches in focus and direction.

Snapshot A: You're driving along a familiar road, so familiar that you begin to daydream. It's only at the last second that you realize you're bearing down on the car in front of you; to avoid a collision, you must jam on the brakes. And you realize that you don't remember any of the drive up till that point; you very likely don't even remember the daydream.

Transforming Stress into Power

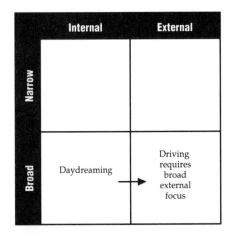

SNAPSHOT A

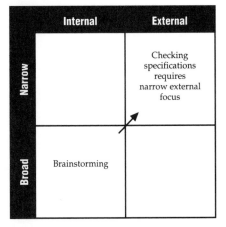

SNAPSHOT B

Driving requires a broad, external focus. You must scan the road, the signs, the pedestrians, the other cars. In this snapshot, you directed your attention broadly but inwardly for your daydream, with near-disastrous results. (Not a bad reminder of just how important attention really is.)

Snapshot B: You're participating successfully and enjoyably in a "brainstorming session" for a major project in your office. Suddenly you're interrupted by an associate who asks you to quickly check the specifications on a proposal she has handed you. You take a quick glance at the numbers and respond, "They look okay." The following week, your boss confronts you with a major error in the specifications. You wonder how you could have overlooked such an obvious error.

Here's where a task, i.e., checking a proposal, requires a narrow external focus: you have to carefully examine all the numbers and letters on the paper. The problem comes when you fail to shift from your broad internal attention (from brainstorming) to the attention necessary for this new task.

Think about the four directions that attention can take, and ask yourself:

- Where would you like to direct more energy in the future?

- Is one direction easier for you than another?

- Where do you presently direct most of your energy?

- Which direction does your spouse, significant other, or best friend prefer?

- What conflicts arise in your relationships as a result of these directional differences?

- Do you find yourself distressed more by the co-worker who frequently seeks to engage you in conversation, or the one who remains quiet and rarely interacts with others?

- What are the most common attention mistakes that you make?

- When a task requires a different type of attention, can you easily make the appropriate shift?

Energy Directors realize that each different situation demands a different intensity and/or focus of attention. They understand that even though each person has a strong *tendency* to prefer one approach toward handling life's problems over another, no one is locked into a tunnel-vision mode. With conscious effort, we are capable of changing the direction of our energy as the need arises; in fact, we *must* do so if we want to be able to clearly plot our way through life.

Getting on Target

In mathematics, a vector is defined as a force or velocity having magnitude and direction. It is usually represented as a line drawn from its origin to its final position. Vectors have a distinct starting and ending point. And the process of getting from one place to another is equally clear; it is straight and true.

Getting on target in life is a little more complicated, for the path between points isn't always so straightforward. How do you achieve direction in your life? Energy Directors do it three ways: through *goals, values, and action.*

Setting Goals

The mind is a goal-oriented system. Goals clarify your purpose and, along with your values, help you to act appropriately. By setting goals, you give your mind the ability to *focus*, which will get you going in the right direction.

We have different goals for different purposes: short-term and long-term goals—goals for getting through the day, and goals for the future. Most of us are able to set the short-term ones, such as what we'll accomplish today, but we tend to have more trouble looking at the long term— where we are heading, say, five, 10, or 15 years from now. (In this way personal planning often parallels North American corporate planning: it focuses on the short-term.) On the following page, you'll find a short exercise to help change your perspective.

Take 15 Minutes to Give Your Life Direction

If you're like 95% of the population, you've never set lifetime goals. In a twenty-five year follow-up study on goal setting, researchers found that 5% of the participants who had set long-term goals lived more fulfilled, successful, and happy lives than those who didn't. Here's your chance to establish goals to give direction to your life's energies. It takes just 15 minutes and three sheets of paper.

Head the first sheet: "My Lifetime Goals." Now, for the next five minutes, write all the things you'd like to do, own, learn, or experience in your life. Go for quantity. List places you'd like to visit; things you want to accomplish; relationships you want to build. What will make your life worth living? Write fast for five full minutes.

Now, on another sheet headed "My Five-Year Goals," list all the things you want to achieve, experience, learn, and acquire over the next five years. Take five minutes, and again, go for quantity.

On a third page headed "My Six-Month Goals," list all the things you'd do if you only had six months to live. How would you live your last six months of life on earth?

Now look at all three lists. Do the five-year goals build toward your lifetime goals? How about the six-month list? Are you living life right now in a way that is consistent with your long-term goals? Are you directing your energy toward your desired future? Try selecting several of the most important items from your lifetime goals and work backwards by determining what short-term and intermediate goals could help you stay on track.

In setting your goals, remember these key points:

- A goal should be written down, first in pencil, then later in ink. This crystallizes your intentions. Make certain you write a positive statement such as: "I am," "I have completed," as opposed to "I would like," or "I will accomplish."

- Make your goal specific and measurable.

- Determine whether you will need the support of others. Some of us can be the Lone Ranger, others need coaches, cheerleaders, and people who believe in us and will remind and support us.

- Rate your commitment to your goal. On a scale of one to ten, how committed are you to the goal? If you can't honestly rate your commitment an "8" or better, rewrite it.

- Keep track of your progress. Do something every day that moves you toward your goal. Ask yourself in which direction you are heading—toward your goal, or away from it?

Energy Directors *do* see themselves as powerful people, able to act upon and transform their lives. They bring to the present a history of small and large successes, which are the results of setting both short- and long-term goals and achieving them.

Understanding Your Values

Victor Frankel, a noted psychiatrist imprisoned in the Nazi prison camps in Germany during WWII, wanted to understand why some people gave up and died while others lived when faced with the same terrifying circumstances. His conclusion was that the survivors lived because they directed their lives with purpose and values. He found four major reasons:

1. They had a sense of lifework or purpose that they were living to fulfill.

2. They had a powerful love of family, and believed they would see their spouses and children at some time in the future.

3. They had a belief in the rightness of the principles of their nation, a sense of patriotism and the importance of freedom.

4. Finally, they had a profound belief in God. By being in touch with the spiritual, they believed they would survive.

Frankel called this "man's search for meaning." These people understood and believed in their values, those that created their purpose and direction—and, in this case, saved their lives.

Transforming Stress into Power

An Exercise in Understanding Your Values

In the space below, we have listed a number of commonly held values. You'll also find some space to add other values that are important to you. Now here comes the fun part. If you had 100 units of energy to spend on *your* values, how would you divide them, according to how important each is to you?

VALUE	ENERGY	VALUE	ENERGY
Truth		Health	
Harmony		Honesty	
Work		World Peace	
Family			
Relationships			
Self-development			
Devotion			
Environment			

Clarifying your values is an important energy-directing step. But the real power comes when your actions are consistent with these values.

Getting Your Actions in Synch With Your Values

One of our favorite stories demonstrates the importance of acting in accordance with your beliefs. In the late forties, the renowned Indian pacifist Mahatma Gandhi represented his country's desires for sovereignty to the British Parliament. Gandhi spoke eloquently and passionately on behalf of independence. The audience, accustomed to the drier, more formal presentations of its members, was spellbound. At the conclusion of the speech, the members clustered around Gandhi's secretary to inquire how Gandhi could speak so long, so eloquently, and so flawlessly without notes, charts, and other oratory devices. His press secretary replied that it was "simple." "What Gandhi thinks, says, and does are one. You think one thing. You say a second. You do a third. That's why you need notes to keep track." It's one thing to have good intentions, another to act upon them. In the final analysis, energy direction involves action. What good are the best developed ideas and plans without implementation?

Taking Action

Now let's look at the third energy-directing step, *action*, in which you move toward your goals and do things in harmony with your values. Most of us have more choices then we can comfortably handle—more stimuli, more pulls in more directions. It's not always easy to sort out what to do and where to go. Sometimes our actions are in conflict with our goals and values. Is the way you actually spend your time and energy consistent with what you believe to be important?

Actions Speak Louder than Words: An Exercise

The boxes below each represent the total amount of waking time and energy you have in a week. Apportion this time (by slicing up Box A as in example B) to represent the percent of your time you spend on:

- Work
- Maintaining the household
- Family
- Friends
- Civic activities
- Groups or organizations
- Exercise and wellness
- Hobbies

Hobbies	
Family	
Exercise	
Maintaining the household	
Work	

Box A
Your Present Situation

Box B
Example

Box C
Your Desired Situation

Is there any time left over? Look back at the exercise in which you apportioned your 100 units of energy to your values. Do you find consistency?

Participants in our seminars are often surprised to discover they spend far more time and energy on work than they do on all the other activities combined. Their life looks like example B. Once they become Energy Directors, many resolve to live a better-balanced life by focusing more efficiently so that they can get more done at work in less time. Now, go ahead and reallocate your energy in Box C, the way you'd like to direct it. What actions will you take to actually make this happen?

Identifying Your Action Blocks: Ready-Set-Go

Just as energy has limited value until you transform it into power, your thoughts, ideas, feelings, and dreams are only worth so much until you act on them. There is simply no other way to find out if your thoughts or ideas really work; until you act, you just won't know. Since the notion that you must act before you can succeed is so simple and logical, why don't more people act out their intentions? Because they're blocked from action by their fears.

The following story, told by a manager who had returned from a wilderness teambuilding experience, demonstrates the power of working through a fear and learning to consciously let go of it.

"I'd never climbed a rock before. For the first several hundred feet I felt exhilarated, and then it hit. Sheer terror. I was halfway up this cliff. I couldn't find the next handhold or foothold. All of a sudden I got scared. I envisioned myself falling. My legs started to quiver, you know, that rubber-legged feeling. I could feel the sweat running down my forehead.

Then, from somewhere out of the blue, I remembered something from a book I had just read. It was a quote from a popular science fiction book called Dune. *There was a scene where a kid has to put his hand in a strange machine called a Gome Jabar. If he gives the wrong answer to a question, he gets zapped and disintegrates. So here he is, like me up on the rock, and he starts repeating this saying over and over to himself:* **I watch the fear come. I watch the fear go. I realize I am not the fear. When the fear leaves, all that will be left is me.**

So I said it three or four times to myself. I could feel my heartbeat slow down, my breathing getting easier. The fear passed. I found my handhold, and I felt the power of working through the fear in my mind.

In this situation, the fear was real—physical danger—yet the greatest obstacle was not the rock but the cold, numbing terror that temporarily paralyzed the climber and prevented him from action. Here are some more common blocks to action that can prevent us from directing our energy appropriately:

The Fear of Commitment

When we make a positive commitment, it motivates, compels, and directs us toward whatever we are committed to. If it is negative, it is mainly seen as a limit on our options and choices. Instead of feeling that we have gained, the feeling is one of loss, of options being closed off, and possibilities limited. Some researchers find that men who remain reluctant to commit to relationships and marriage have been paralyzed by a sense of "what if a better deal comes along?" They fear closing out options and becoming boxed in.

There is a power to commitment—we need to remember that. An exercise we use in our workshops to demonstrate this power goes as follows:

Take a moment to "center yourself" (more about this later) by sitting up straight, getting free from any distractions, removing anything constraining (glasses, shoes). Uncross your legs and arms. If you'd like, you can close your eyes. Take a few deep breaths and imagine the following:

Think about a time and place, either in the past or the present, when you were doing something to which you felt a deep, abiding commitment. Something you believed in fervently and did with a passion. Use all your senses to recall this image. How did it look? Once you have recalled this time, if you had to describe what it was like to someone else, using one word, what would that one word be?

We have conducted this exercise with thousands of people; they have described their experiences with words like: *energized, powerful, content, tranquil, serene, loving, happy, fulfilled.* And the list goes on and on. Compare these

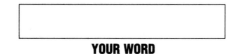

YOUR WORD

Transforming Stress into Power

words to the terms you would use to describe a *lack* of commitment. Which feelings would you rather experience?

Fear of Change

Why do most people resist change? Probably because they believe in the saying, "The devil you know is better than the devil you don't know." The present situation with its limitations and shortcomings may be better than the unknown. They are concerned about upsetting the familiar and the comfortable.

Successful changes often upset a delicate balance, particularly in relationships. We will often see this with middle-aged couples. One decides to make a major health improvement (i.e. lose weight or get fit) that the other has trouble adapting to. This one-sided change creates stress within the relationship. In fact, this one issue could drive the couple apart, especially if the other party remains resistant.

Sometimes one successful change leads to a series of other changes. A study focusing on the lives of people who had stopped smoking six months previously found that the new ex-smokers had made all sorts of other changes in their lives. Many had changed jobs, relationships, hobbies; they had moved to new towns and made new friends. After discovering their newfound power, they started "flexing their muscles." "After all," they thought, "If I can quit smoking, I can do just about anything!" That's empowerment!

Fear of Success

It seems strange when you look at it in print, but you'd be amazed at how widespread fear of success is. Changes make people evaluate their links and bonds with others . . . and with themselves. The fear-of-success concept often brings up guilt. The unhappy subject thinks, "Somehow I don't deserve to be: A) happy, B) successful, C) in love, D) all of the above. After all, none of my friends are."

One way of breaking through the barrier of negative self-dialog is by affirming the positive. An affirmation is a conscious, positive statement or image that channels your energy into action. It can be a written statement, something you repeat to yourself, or it can be an internal or external picture—a vision of yourself being successful or a picture of the ideal goal on your refrigerator. If your attachment to your block is strong, or has been there for a while, you may feel a little uncomfortable with the affirmation. Stay with it. When you catch yourself feeling that "you don't deserve success," try repeating some of the following phrases to yourself:

"I deserve success."

"Success is mine now."

"I am happy, fulfilled, prosperous, and successful."

"It is natural for me to succeed."

"I've studied, prepared, and worked for success."

Fear of Failure

Fear of failure is even more common than fear of success. "What if my entrepreneurial business doesn't make it?" "What if I can't quit smoking?" "What if I can't lose weight?" The dilemma is that we often measure and evaluate ourselves through the eyes of others: "What if I don't make it? Will I look silly?"

Energy Directors train themselves to look at failures as learning experiences. Thomas Edison, for example, figured out 10,000 ways to *not* make light come from electricity moving through a filament...but only one successful light bulb.

Lack of Motivation

This is actually a two-part problem: 1) getting started, and 2) continuing to move. One approach we use in our workshops to help participants initiate action is an exercise in visualization. We ask the participants to imagine that a Genie magically appears and grants them total power—in whatever they choose to do, they will achieve total success. We then ask, "If you knew you would not fail, what would you do? How would your life be different? What new enterprises would you start? What would be different day in and day out?"

Continuing to move once we've started is another issue. One of the most common barriers is setting unrealistic goals and, after not having achieved them, beating ourselves up psychologically by whittling away at our self-esteem. We hear comments like "I have no will power," or, "I'm a failure." The secret of change is to break things down to bite-sized goals and experience many frequent successes. Why? First, so you get to celebrate frequently. Second, so you reinforce the belief that you are a powerful person who is in control, who can make things happen, who can act upon and transform your life.

The Lack of Role Models

Many people don't have the opportunity to work or be with others who are successful, achieving, and getting results in their lives. "If you hang out with turkeys, how can you expect to soar like an eagle?" goes the contemporary saying, containing a truth we all recognize. We learn success, effective action, and power by being with others who are successful, effective, and powerful. If you don't know any people with these characteristics, start searching for some.

Read biographies of great successes, profiles of entrepreneurs, articles on how others are succeeding in their fields or professions. Make a list of the most successful people you know in your own profession. Call one with an invitation to lunch. Tell the person you admire his or her success (who doesn't like to be admired?) and would like to hear firsthand how it was achieved. Make a career move to place yourself on winning teams or in companies with winning products or services. Scout out the best coach or mentor you can find to learn from.

Do you recognize any of these blocks as your own? Can you add any to the list? If you're busy blocking your own progress, how can you summon the energy necessary for growth? Energy Directors keep the "big picture" in mind. Unlike people who "can't see the forest for the trees," they know what's important, they overcome blocks, and they go for it. **You** can be one of them.

Just three steps are necessary to transform your potential into energy and success: **goals**, **values**, and **action**. Now all that's missing is the knowledge and skill to apply them. In chapters 5-8, we will be covering ways to develop your grounding, creative, logic, and relationship energies. As you read through these chapters, please do so with the idea of using these techniques to better direct your life—toward your goals, and in synch with your values.

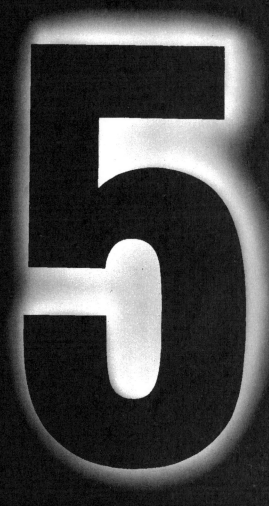

GROUNDING
ENERGY

Grounding Energy

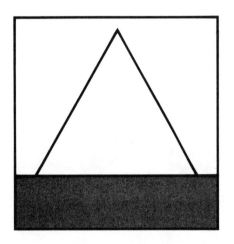

As we learned in Chapter 3, there are four types of energy in our lives. And people with dominance in each category exhibit unique abilities.

What highly grounded people do best is to constantly utilize their senses to get information about the world around them. They have an awareness of the external and internal world based upon these senses.

Grounding energy is all about the present moment. People who are highly grounded achieve full awareness as their senses function in the here and now. If you are strong in this energy, the present moment is not robbed by your mind jumping ahead into future possibilities or options, nor are you pulled back by strong emotions or feelings from the past. When you use grounding energy, you pick up on the cues and clues that life provides daily. If you were attracted by the cover of this book, your senses were working for you.

What do you get from using your senses? Information—about the world around you, about other people, and about how things work. This is information or feedback that's a crucial trigger for the other energies. Creative, logic, and relationship energies depend upon good input. Your actions are ordered and colored by the use of your senses. Grounding energy, fed by your senses, adds a practical, tangible, realistic flavor to all that you do.

Transforming Stress into Power

People who are highly grounded have a "penchant for action." They tend to be extremely practical and realistic, and learn best by doing, trying, and repeating.

An Awareness of the Senses

Our physical senses: seeing, touching, tasting, smelling, and hearing help us gather data from the world. This physical awareness connects us with the "present moment" by grounding us in the here-and-now.

Highly grounded individuals are at one extreme: when they're out walking, they notice the wind on their face, the shadows on the ground, the subtle color differences of the leaves, the smell of grass, trees, and shrubbery, the sounds the birds and other animals are making.

At the other extreme is the person who is so inner-directed, so high in creative energy, and so low in grounding energy that he or she rarely notices anything in the external environment. A good example is the creatively energized psychologist colleague of ours who recently had new furniture installed in his office. His associates took bets on how many days would pass before he noticed the changes. To no one's surprise, it took him three days.

How Grounded Are You?

Count the number of letter F's in the following sentence. (See page 68 for the answer.)

FINISHED FILES ARE THE RESULT OF YEARS OF SCIENTIF-IC STUDY COMBINED WITH THE EXPERIENCE OF MANY YEARS.

How Sensory Information is Received

We all have preferred ways of bringing sensory information in and learning from it. Probably 85% of all people learn visually; the phrases "Draw me a picture," and "I won't believe it until I see it," reflect this strong preference. This sort of person is drawn to the pictures, illustrations, and charts in this book.

The second largest group learns auditorily—*listening* for both the content and the emotional tone of the message. These are the people who listen to tapes in their car, or who would rather listen to this book on audio than read it. It's as if they have a tape recorder in their heads. All they have to do is "rewind the tape," and they can play back mentally anything they've heard.

A very small percentage of people learn best through their tactile, or kinesthetic, senses. Their hands have to hold, turn, or shape an object to know it. "Let me get the feel of it" is their favorite saying. When it comes to learning a sport, dance, or a craft, they can't just read or hear about it, they have to *do* it.

People who concentrate on developing more grounding energy are able to more fully utilize and develop *all* their senses, instead of relying on only one.

Stress: Closing Down the Senses

Have you ever noticed that when you are stressed, you miss or overlook things? Several years ago, we did a study at a major electronics company to find out why there was an increased number of auto accidents right before the Christmas Holidays. We interviewed accident victims and asked them what was happening in the moments immediately preceding their accident. We found that they were internally distracted by strong feelings—either positive (such as looking forward to the visit of an in-law), or negative (looking forward to the visit of an in-law). These strong feelings shut down their senses and affected their ability to drive safely. In short, they weren't functioning in the present moment. Strong emotions upset their ability to react to external stimuli by pulling them out of the present moment.

Forces Coming at Us

We live in a world of multiple stimuli; there's just too much going on in the world for us to be aware of every single stimulus. Psychologists know that the Reticular Activating System (RAS) at the base of the brain continuously filters stimuli from the outer environment. Some input is allowed to enter your mind's awareness, some is not. For example, when you first turn on your computer you may notice, and perhaps be irritated by, the sound of the fan humming, but in a few moments you won't even notice that sound because the RAS has filtered out this continuous stimulation. Without the ability to filter out the stimuli we don't need, we'd be overwhelmed in no time.

Problems occur when we begin to filter out input that we need in order to act appropriately. And when do we do that? When we're under extreme stress. We lose track of details; things become fuzzy; we cease to be aware of others' points of view or how we are coming across to them. We no longer gather the information we really need to solve problems and capitalize on opportunities.

Energy Directors quickly realize when their awareness is blocked or limited. They notice when their perception is

---

Answer to Grounding Quiz on page 67

Did you find the 6 letter F's in the sentence?

Finished Files are the result oF years oF scientiFic study combined with the experience oF many years.

If so, you undoubtedly used grounding energy to carefully notice each letter.

Transforming Stress into Power

narrowing, or becoming fuzzy, and they take the necessary steps to open up their world. They make an effort to bring in, and focus on, new stimuli in order to renew and refresh themselves.

When you experience a shutdown of your senses, you need to develop a plan, exercise, or a "ritual" to pull you back into the moment and regain touch with the here and now. This grounding, or ritual, serves as an organizing principle—a stable center around which you revolve and begin to build other activities.

Grounding Rituals: Tools for Centering Yourself

We once had an opportunity to make a major presentation to the board of directors of a large Wall Street brokerage firm, and to sit in on a decision-making meeting involving a seven-figure financial commitment. The principals each logically expressed the pros and cons of the proposal and examined both the big-picture ramifications and the nitty-gritty details. Finally, after ten minutes of discussion, the decision was left for the chairman to make.

The chairman then reached into his pocket for a well-worn pipe, into another pocket for a pouch of tobacco, and into a third pocket for one of those all-in-one pipe cleaning tools. As the directors watched in silence and anticipation, he used the tool to clean out the stem of the pipe, opened the pouch, took several pinches of tobacco that he pushed into the bowl of the pipe, and tamped down with the tool. Grasping the bowl firmly in one hand, he lit the pipe with a packet of matches, leaned back in his chair, took a long, (it seemed like forever) slow puff, and exhaled, filling the room with a pungent, cinnamon-like odor. Finally, he seemed to almost squeeze the bowl three or four more times, and then he rendered his opinion.

In the example of the Wall Street chairman, unfortunately, the grounding ritual—fondling and lighting a pipe—is associated with a negative health habit. For many people, smoking is a form of ritual; they use it for pacing and for collecting themselves, i.e., "When I finish this cigarette, I'll start on the next problem," or, "I'll think about this over a cigarette." There are many other grounding devices available, with many fewer side effects.

Find a grounding ritual that works for you. Here are some common ones:

Grounding Rituals

- Write with a special pen and paper

- Fondle a smooth stone

- Listen to music

- Clean the house

- Straighten the closets

- Take a brisk walk

- Enjoy a hot bath

- Stretch

- Touch jewelry (twist a ring, fiddle with a chain, etc.)

- Take a coffee break

- Gaze at a favorite picture

- Tend to plants

- Play with a two-year-old

Feel free to add your own special ritual to the list...and make certain to use it to help ground your energy and center yourself.

Exercise and Nutrition: The Primers of Grounding

Some of the best forms of grounding involve physical activity and nutrition. Both are training grounds for sensory awareness and offer the added benefit of providing energy.

Physical energy is the foundation for your energy system. When it is high, it can boost the other systems; when you are in shape, your self-esteem (the emotional relationship

Transforming Stress into Power

you have with yourself) is increased, and you can think more clearly. Physical energy enhances all the other energies, and a lack of it detracts from them. Pain, illness, fatigue, exhaustion can all zap your strength. They cause you to be depressed, to be unable to focus, to relate to others, or to think things through. Ask yourself how much work you get done when you're not feeling well.

Your Personal Environment

Your own sensory awareness begins with your very "personal" environment—your physical fitness. When you are fit, you "see and feel" (i.e., sense) the physical tension in a muscle. You appreciate the strength as that muscle contracts. You know the difference between tension and relaxation. You experience the "high" that comes with aerobic training, the light, clear sensation as your body kicks into a higher level of performance by attending to its physical need for activity. You become empowered.

A participant in one of our workshops told us the story of why he took up jogging. He was at a point in his life when there was a great deal of chaos at home and at work. Two weeks after moving, his family suffered a major flood in the basement. A week after that, his wife lost her job. The same week, his boss left and his whole department was without a sense of direction while the company searched for a successor.

Our participant took up jogging—not for any particular health benefit, but to regain some control over his life. There were so many factors in his life that he couldn't control, but for thirty minutes a day, while jogging, he was in charge! All he had to do was to put one foot in front of the other.

Regular aerobic exercises, those that move the major muscles of the body in a sustained fashion (such as brisk walking, jogging, swimming, and biking), can provide you with the endurance, efficiency, and effectiveness you need if you want to move to higher levels of personal power.

Aerobic conditioning delivers a whole payload of benefits: It strengthens the cardiovascular system, makes weight loss more effective, and helps you look and feel better. To gain these benefits, you'll want to exercise for 30 minutes a session, three to five times a week, taking care not to overstrain. Make certain you can carry on a normal conversation while exercising, and never get short of breath.

Aerobic activity, and exercise in general, provides another benefit: it gets you in touch with your senses. You *feel* the wind on your face, *notice* the sweat, *sense* tendons stretching and muscles contracting.

Exercise is a balance for highly creative people. Often, they will start out with their minds racing for the first ten, fifteen, or twenty minutes; then, if the aerobic period is long enough, they get in a groove where they no longer avoid or shut out the sensations from their body. Their creative energy takes on a more grounded nature; their normal burst-like impulsive energy becomes more constant. Their minds relax as they focus in the here-and-now. Later they will often find a fresh source of creative inspiration because they can approach their work in a new way.

Good Nutrition and Energy

As they say, "You can't have one without the other." No matter how high you prove to be in a certain energy, you can't capitalize on that energy if you're fueling your body with junk food.

Your body needs a solid energy base to work with. It gets that energy from three food sources: proteins, fats, and carbohydrates. Not all those sources provide the same number of energy units (calories). A gram of fat, for instance, produces nine calories of energy when burned in your body as fuel; a gram of protein or carbohydrate only produces about four and a half calories.

"Oh, that's great," we hear you saying. "Now I have a good excuse for eating only high-fat foods like ice cream and chips—I'll have more energy." Well, think again.

Fat may contain energy, but its drawbacks far outweigh its advantages: it can raise our cholesterol level and clog our arteries; it contributes to weight gain; and it may be responsible for the high occurrence of certain kinds of cancer (e.g. colon, breast). Also, while fat may provide more energy units than other food sources, our bodies take longer to digest high-fat foods than foods high in

Transforming Stress into Power

proteins and carbohydrates. And the ability to digest fat decreases with age.

Stoking Your Body's Furnace

People today are eating a diet far too heavy in fat: 42% of the calories we consume come from that source, even though experts suggest that the ideal healthy diet should consist of only about 30% fat. We aren't suggesting that you give up fats altogether. We simply urge that you adjust your diet so that complex carbos and proteins (those based on whole grains) become the "hardwood" of your energy's fire (we'll allow you an occasional "log" of fat), and that you relegate sugar to the role of "kindling."

A True "Power Lunch"

Are you a victim of the 2 p.m. energy slump? Your lunch may be the culprit. Research has proven that a high-protein, low-fat meal can increase mental alertness. This translates to a lunch menu that avoids or minimizes non-diet mayonnaise, creamy salad dressings, buttery sauces, and anything breaded or fried.

The following suggestions for more "thought-provoking" lunch items are not revolutionary, but they are low in fats and high in ingredients that will increase your mental energy level:

*A main dish, salad, or sandwich made from skinless poultry, fish, or lean meat (or eggs, but no more than 3-4 per week)...on

*Whole wheat bread, a whole grain roll, or pita...OR

*Low fat yogurt or cottage cheese

These dishes can be accompanied by fresh fruits and vegetables which, while not particularly contributing to mental energy, will provide variety and flavor, and will certainly not detract from it.

The sort of quickly digested lunch we just described contains protein-based chemicals that will energize your brain for its afternoon's work—letting you direct your energy outward. Isn't that better than feeling mentally sluggish from 1 until 4 while trying to digest a high-fat, high-sugar meal?

In addition to exercise and nutrition, there are other ways to increase your grounding energy.

● **Do one thing at a time.**

Resist the temptation to become scattered. Ask yourself at the beginning of the day, "What is it I want to accomplish?" Then stay focused to achieve it. Ask yourself, "What is the best use of my energy right now?" Then take your own advice.

● **Eat a sensuous meal.**

The next time you eat a meal, slow down and fully experience the sights, textures, tastes, and smells of the food. To understand this concept, imagine that you are a prisoner about to be executed and, as your last request, you have been granted the meal of your choice. It is the very last meal you'll ever eat. How would you eat this meal using all your senses, recognizing that the more you notice, the more you attend, the longer you'll live, and the more you'll enjoy your food?

● **Use a visual centering device.**

A mandala is a pattern that includes a center with forms radiating from it. (A snowflake is an example of a typical mandala-like form.) You draw upon grounding energy when focusing your attention on such a pattern, and it can have a calming and orderly effect on you. In our office, oriental rugs serve this purpose.

● **Think of your body as a testing ground.**

Modifying your routines will force you to become more aware of the world around you. Keep a diary that details the effects of caffeine, food, stretching, and exercise on your energy, attitude, and mood. Change your diet for a week (give up sweets, eliminate meat, eat more pasta, etc.). Take up meditation. Get up an hour earlier. In short, disrupt the patterns that have lulled you into sensory oblivion.

● **Get "out of your head" and in touch with your hands.**

Take up a hobby that requires you to use your hands. Try knitting, gardening, building model airplanes, fixing cars, or doing home fix-up projects—anything that causes you to increase your awareness of your hands and your sense of touch.

- **Put your body into a position of power.**

  Physical power comes from body image and alignment; energy moves more efficiently through a correctly aligned body. Spend some time observing peoples' postures. Select a few different postures. Put your body into each position, and become aware of how it feels. Right now, move your body into a position that gives you a feeling of power.

- **Ask grounding questions.**

  Develop the habit of asking "Do I have all the information I need? What other information could I get by listening, looking, touching, tasting, or smelling?" Information gathering is not just a passive process of sitting and waiting; you have to go out and get it. Ask questions, explore, manipulate objects. Watch people in a store and see which displays attract their attention.

- **Celebrate your accomplishments frequently.**

  Take time to celebrate your little successes. Enjoy the feeling of completion. Build "finish lines," and rewards into your daily routine.

- **Get a massage.**

  A full body massage is a good way to get in touch with your body. In addition to feeling great, it can help you find the tight spots where you tend to accumulate tension. Thirty or fifty minutes on the table will force you to slow down and experience your body.

- **Take three deep breaths.**

  No matter where you are or how busy you are, you have time to take three deep breaths. Do this every few hours, or whenever you feel tension catching up with you. Breathe in slowly and deeply. Do not raise your shoulders, but let your abdomen expand as you inhale and contract as you exhale. Feel tension leaving your body as the air flows out of your lungs. Repeat at least twice.

Grounding Energy

- ## Use autosuggestion.

One way to get in better touch with your body is to provide it with autosuggestions. These act as commands that help to calm nervous and muscular activity. Repeat the following to yourself:

Autosuggestion Commands

I feel quiet.

I am beginning to feel relaxed.

My whole body feels comfortable and relaxed.

My hands are warm and relaxed.

My mind is calm and quiet.

- ## Feel the difference between tension and relaxation.

A good exercise to increase awareness of your body involves systematically tensing and relaxing your muscles. Lie down. Loosen your clothing and do the following: Tighten the muscles in your right foot. Squeeze hard for a count of three, then relax the muscles completely. Now do the same with your left foot. Gradually work your way up your body, alternatively tensing and then relaxing all your muscle groups: legs, abdomen, back, hands, arms, shoulders, neck, and face. Fully experience the difference between tension and relaxation. Also, realize and appreciate how comfortable you now feel. This is a great exercise for getting the tension out of your body so that you can sleep at night.

- ## The last suggestion.

We've enjoyed the contribution highly grounded people make to our workshops (and to our organization). When the creative types are off in outer space, the analysts are paralyzed with decision-making, and the relationship people are overwhelmed by feelings, the highly grounded people save the day. Their message is crisp and clear: "Let's just do it."

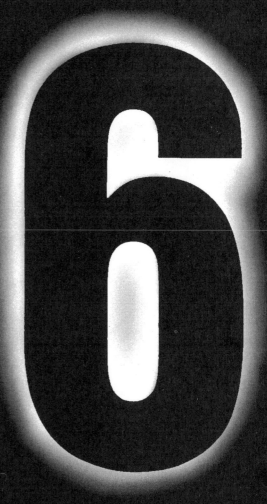

CREATIVE
ENERGY

Creative Energy

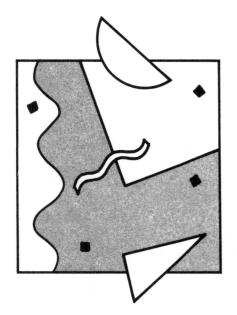

".. .I look at what has never been, and say, 'Why not?'"
The famous John F. Kennedy quote, whether Kennedy
knew it or not, is a classic example of creative energy.
Creative energy takes us into the future and into
possibilities not dreamt before. It's the ability to look at a
situation or problem and come up with multiple
"What if. . ." approaches to a solution. Often it gives us
funny and even bizarre looks at the ordinary; it can come
to us in the form of a "Eureka!"-type flash of inspiration,
or it can provide us with the solution in bits and pieces.
Creative energy, in short, is the ability to tap into the mind
at play—and if that sounds like fun, it is.

Naturally, not everybody sees it that way. If you were
ever scolded in school for daydreaming, letting your mind
wander, searching for something more interesting than
your class—your teacher was discounting your creative
energy. The problem is that in our development, creativity
may have gotten quashed. Children quickly learn that
there is only one right answer to a question.

Everyone has creative energy and the potential to develop
it. Many of us have much more than we think.

Creative Energy is a Part of Your Everyday Life

Look around your room right now. Everything in the room was, at one time, someone's creative idea: your furniture, your tools, the pictures on the wall. Each was once an inventive solution, even an inspiration, different than any solution or inspiration before it.

We receive creative messages in many ways and in many forms. Fantasies and daydreams are common sources. Dreams at night have often solved problems that their dreamers have been working on consciously for weeks, months, sometimes years. Creative solutions can just as easily sneak into our awareness while we're doing something totally unrelated: doodling on a sheet of paper, singing in the shower, working out.

It's Not Just for Artists

The first important fact to learn about creativity is that it's not the sole province of writers, artists, sculptors, or poets. Except for the most menial tasks, almost every form of useful work requires creative energy. Creative energy is used by the business person, the marketing executive, the engineer, the newspaper columnist, the homemaker, the machinist, the caseworker, and the secretary. We use its tools in our work every day; it offers ways to open up problems and discover solutions. It's absolutely essential for breaking out of our distress-producing ruts.

How do we tap into this wonderful, freewheeling energy? There is a number of techniques, all equally productive; and besides, when it comes to creative energy, anything and everything is possible. The techniques we're going to explore closely include:

- LETTING GO OF LIMITS

- CHANGING PERSPECTIVE

- BRAINSTORMING

- VISUALIZING

- INTUITIVE PROCESSING

Letting Go of Limits

Back in the early 20th century, there was a terrific but wacky baseball player named Germany Schaefer, who simply could not accept the notion that the earth revolved on its axis. To prove his point, he filled the bathtub with water each night and explained to his doubters, "If we were goin' 'round, how come the water don't slosh out on the floor?"

The point is that each of us lives in a world that is limited by our experience and beliefs. These limits make us feel secure; they make the world seem stable and regular. In Columbus' day, most people believed the world was flat; and not only was there the danger of sailing off the edge, but what was one to do about all those horrid sea serpents? No wonder Columbus had to go all the way to the Queen to find a sponsor for his explorations.

For decades, everyone believed that a four-minute mile was the absolute limit of how fast a person could run. Obviously, Roger Bannister, who was the first to break the barrier, did not subscribe to that belief—and his record has since been battered by almost twenty seconds! Bannister, Columbus, the Wright Brothers, and countless others are examples of people who simply did not share the limiting beliefs of the day.

Limiting Beliefs

Here are a few common limiting beliefs. Do you recognize any as your own?

"We can't."

"It's impossible."

"I'm too old."

"It's never been done before."

"I'm not that kind of person."

"No one can do that."

Take a sheet of paper and write down some of your own often-used limiting beliefs. Then go ahead and make a paper airplane out of your list. Toss the plane out the window. Or wad the paper up, pretend it's a basketball, and shoot it into a wastebasket. Free yourself of these limitations. Let your imagination soar, and score two points for creativity.

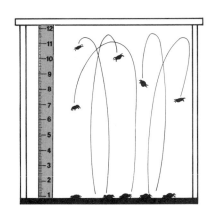

Imagine for a moment the following: Place 100 fleas in a large box, 12" deep. On the top of the box, place a glass lid. Now watch as the fleas start jumping. Without the lid each would jump several feet. They quickly start banging their heads against the glass. After a few moments they start adjusting the height of their jumps to 11 7/8 inches. Soon the entire flea circus is jumping just short of the glass top. Now remove the glass. What happens? The fleas remain in the box, each jumping just 11 7/8 inches, no more.

The fascinating thing about creative energy is that it knows no limits. It's not constrained by time, place, or practicality. It's the energy of intuition; it just takes off and soars. If you have no sensory data about a problem, this is the only energy that will solve it; and of course you cannot touch, smell, or gather information about the future in any other way.

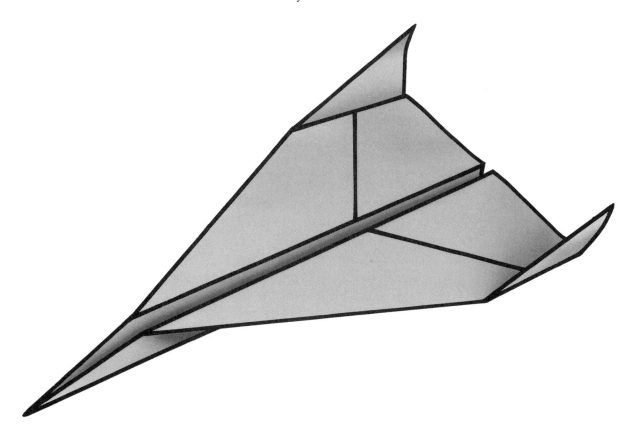

Changing Your Perspective

Consider a problem you're stuck on right now. It could be the new advertising campaign; it could be a way to reverse a slipping sales curve; it could be a procedure to make your files more accessible. Whatever it is, if you're stuck for a solution, we'll bet, sight unseen, that you're looking at it from only one point of view. Why do that, when you've already proved that it's not working? Try looking at your problem from these perspectives:

- How would you explain it to a five-year old? To someone who doesn't speak your language? To a visitor from another planet?

- Imagine the problem as an object. What shape and color would it be? What would it look like if you made it bigger? Smaller? Out of another material? Turned it upside down? Inside out? Backwards or sideways?

- How would Einstein, or any of *your* favorite creative thinkers, look at this?

- If you could leap 20 years ahead and look back on the problem and a solution, how would it seem?

- If someone else is waiting for your solution, how do you suppose the problem looks to that person?

Of course, there are no hard-and-fast techniques to be applied to every situation that arises. The point is just the opposite: *there are no limits to possibilities and perspectives, except the ones you impose yourself.* Each different look you take at a problem and its solutions offers you something you're not seeing from your present perspective.

The perspective you have today is but one of millions available to you, but if you're really stuck on a problem, that single perspective happens to be one that offers no solutions. By all means try another one. Over several days (assuming you have that much time), develop and list as many perspectives and solutions as you can. Then go back and look at the different possibilities and see how they might be combined or put to work. Chances are you'll find a solution...or even more than one.

Brainstorming

Originally conceived almost 50 years ago as a group function, this works on an individual level too. Brainstorming is a technique requiring concentration on the present situation, the goal being to build upon each other's (or your own) ideas. The ideal number for a group is five to 10 participants.

Brainstorming got its name because each person in the group is asked to use his or her brain to attack a creative problem in the manner of commandos storming an objective. But if you're willing to open up your imagination, you can accomplish the same things on your own.

Guidelines for Brainstorming

1. The group (or you) agrees to suspend all judgment. No idea is wrong, silly, dumb, impractical, or impossible. There will be time enough to criticize later, but not now.

2. Wildness is welcome, the more off-the-wall the better.

3. Whether it's an individual or group session, everyone involved knows clearly what the problem is that needs solving.

4. Decide how long the session will last or else the session will ramble on and become boring and uncomfortable, if not incoherent. The ideal time is 20 to 30 minutes, no longer.

5. Go for quantity. In brainstorming, more is better.

6. Build upon others' (or, if it's just you, the preceding) ideas and suggestions. Rule nothing out; everybody's contributions are of worth.

7. Write the ideas on a chart pack or a blackboard so that everyone can see them all at the same time. In a group, a leader is needed who will maintain the ground rules and see that all ideas are recorded and that the session ends on time.

Here are some other "brainstorming-type" activities that you can easily do alone:

● Put Together an Idea Notebook

Creative people find that ideas come at odd and unexpected times. For people who are not accustomed to tapping their creative energy, we suggest a couple of methods useful to capture creative ideas. First, start an idea notebook. Keep it with you at all times. When you have a new idea, jot it down. Keep the book by your bed so that if you wake up with some creative ideas you will have it handy. We know of one scientist who has catalogued over 14,000 creative ideas this way through the years. He uses them to develop ideas for his research endeavors and in his scientific writings.

Creativity can come from others and from life itself. Anton Chekov, the famous Russian writer, always kept a phrase notebook with him. When people in his life would say something interesting or describe unique situations, he would note them in his book. After collecting notebooks filled with hundreds of quotes, situations, and pieces of information, he would weave these into the characters in his stories and plays. He tapped into the real world to generate ideas and create variations of words, themes, and content for his work.

If writing is not for you, carry a small tape recorder with you. When you have a creative idea, stop at that moment and dictate it into the recorder. Keep adding ideas, concepts, hunches, whatever seems interesting. When you have filled a tape, transcribe it, or listen to it for inspiration.

Next, use the ideas from your notebook or tape as the "stuff" for creating. Start clustering and forming these fragments into larger concepts and more developed notions.

● Do a Brain Dump

From computer technology we have learned how to "dump" at one time all that is stored in a computer file or memory. So just sit down and start dumping onto paper all the ideas you have about a particular topic. Jot down full ideas, half ideas, half-baked ideas. Keep writing anything that comes to mind. Go for a complete dump of everything you know about that subject. Just keep forcing yourself to generate content, concepts, insights, feelings, words, pictures, phrases, and sentences around the topic. Later take the brain dump and look at it. Separate the valuable from the not-so-valuable and use the valuable to build the concept and ideas you are developing.

● Sketch an Idea Molecule

Start by doodling. On a large piece of paper, write a key idea in the middle of the page. This is the seed idea. From that seed start a branch with other ideas. Keep adding them. Use the ideas to generate still more ideas. Come back to the seed idea and start generating another branch. Use this branch to build still more ideas. You are creating an idea molecule that may not build logically—it may grow in sudden jumps and in unexpected ways. Build on the idea molecule with other molecules to create more complete creative products.

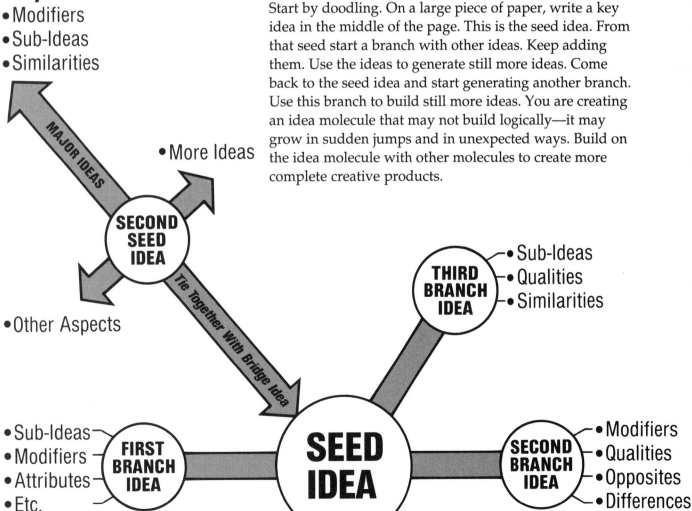

Major Ideas
- Modifiers
- Sub-Ideas
- Similarities

MAJOR IDEAS

- More Ideas

SECOND SEED IDEA

Tie Together With Bridge Idea

- Other Aspects

THIRD BRANCH IDEA
- Sub-Ideas
- Qualities
- Similarities

- Sub-Ideas
- Modifiers
- Attributes
- Etc.

FIRST BRANCH IDEA

SEED IDEA

SECOND BRANCH IDEA
- Modifiers
- Qualities
- Opposites
- Differences

Visualizing

"If you can think it, you can do it." That's the essence of visualizing, a skill that uses your imagination to picture possibilities. It builds upon the ways in which we capture images as pictures in our minds (most memory is visual memory in the form of "snapshots:" a holiday dinner from your childhood, your first-born child, your favorite vacation location). And visualizing allows us to see future possibilities, actions, and scenarios.

Like creative energy itself, visualizing is the free play of the imagination; it is not limited by time, space, practicality, or reality. Visualizing can be used to bring about specific goals. To use the example of basketball, it's well documented that teams have achieved dramatic improvement in their free-throw shooting by having each player invest 20 minutes or so in visualizing successful free throws. The players are asked to close their eyes and imagine the scene: their teammates and opponents lined up on the foul line, the rim and net, the ball in their hands, correct form and release, and the ball swishing cleanly through. In combination with good old-fashioned practice and hard work, this really works.

The technique of visualizing is not only effective in sports but also in public presentations or any other individual effort that you'd like to improve. But it's important that you recognize the difference between visualizing and simply *wishing* that things were so. Visualizing is more focused than that; it's a very real skill that requires practice. Try it on a daily basis and you'll get better at it. Begin each day visualizing the success you will achieve—whatever form that success takes—and the goals you will accomplish. On the following page are some specific steps to take to learn the process.

How Velcro Was Invented

In a creative visualization session, the inventor of Velcro had a fantasy. The inventor visualized a man running through a thicket in a forest. The thorns on the bushes tore at his clothes, leaving small pieces stuck on the branches. Working with the image of thorns and points meeting soft fabric, the Velcro fastener was created. Today we use this material in children's shoes, clothing, and an assortment of bags. From this one fantasy grew a multi-million dollar company.

Transforming Stress into Power

Five Steps for Visualizing

1. Allow yourself absolute permission to do nothing but visualize—that is, imagine—for the next 10 to 20 minutes.

2. Find a quiet space, free from interruptions or distractions (not always easy, but a must), and sit in a comfortable position. Take off your glasses, loosen or remove restricting clothing, and close your eyes.

3. Take several deep breaths and allow your body to relax.

4. Rub the palms of your hands together until they are good and warm. Cup your palms over your eyes, shutting out all light. Let your eyelashes brush your palms.

5. Look up slightly with your eyes and begin to see the images you want to see in your mind. Imagine solutions with your mind. Play with images and combinations. Allow the "movie screen in your mind" to generate an unusual daydream or story to solve the problem.

Intuitive Processing

Hunches come at different times and different places, but at one time or another we've all had them. They have to do with our seeing the results of a new idea. Research has shown that hunches often occur in activities in which our concentration is focused on something else altogether.

People who are skilled with creative energy will learn to take walks, work out, take a shower or a nap, ride a bike—anything that doesn't require massive focused concentration and that will let them open up to their creative power. When that happens, they've successfully shifted their focus inward to a broad mode of concentration, and the intuitive process can take over.

Many creative people have awakened in the morning with a clear picture of the answer to the problem they were wrestling with the day before; it's not uncommon to wake up in the wee hours with an entire stream of ideas, each containing possible solutions. Although people usually stumble over this marvelous process the first time, it's well-researched, and experts at it can put it to work whenever they choose.

How to Tap Your Intuition

1. "Program" the problem the night before so that your creative energy can get to work on it.

2. Write the problem down clearly on a piece of paper by your bed.

3. Tell yourself that when you awaken, you'll know the solution to the problem.

4. When you wake up, scribble the very first ideas that come to mind.

5. Use those answers later.

There's no limit to the sorts of cues your intuition can pick up on and put to creative use; anything from your private universe (the totality of your conscious and unconscious experiences) can be tapped into. Creative energy is everywhere.

The eminent Swiss psychiatrist Dr. Carl Jung found that when people really open themselves to creative energy, the creativity process draws from more than just their conscious efforts. The creative process can even generate, for example, the familiar occurrences we know as "deja vu."

Have you ever experienced "deja vu," in which you find yourself in a situation that seems identical to one you encountered in the past? Creative people who are open to suggestion can use such a coincidence, called *synchronicity*, to draw on the past for help with their present situation.

Have you ever been working, for example, on a creative problem, and then taken a break, opened a book, talked with a friend, or even (Heaven forbid) turned on the TV and—lo and behold—there's the same topic being discussed, or some information that just fits the idea you've been struggling with? The key to tapping into these synchronistic events is to be open and aware.

Transforming Stress into Power

Turn on Creativity by Doing Something Symbolic

Have you ever had a creativity block? Been stopped dead in your creative tracks? Felt that your creativity had dried up? Found that none of your old techniques for reviving it worked? Almost all artists, writers, scientists, and business people who must tap their creative energy for a living occasionally experience this "stress panic."

How can you get past a creative block crisis? You might try some symbolic activities to turn on your creativity. Plant a garden: dig in the earth and turn the soil; throw out the stones and pull the weeds. Plant some seeds. Water them and sit with your creativity tools, watching and waiting. Be patient. Soon, will find shoots of green in the garden and shoots of ideas in your mind. Nurture the garden and nurture the new ideas.

If gardening doesn't appeal to you, redo a room, make a quilt—undertake any project from scratch in which your own physical labor creates a pleasing result. Then move on to your "mental" labor—your creative work. You'll find that your creative energy has been renewed.

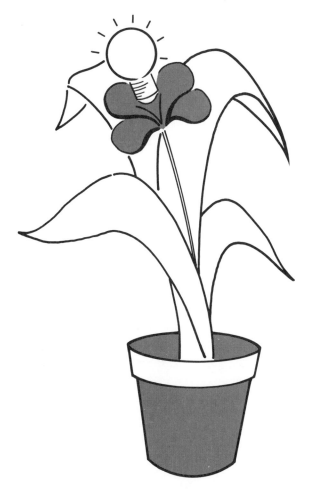

Need still more ideas? Creative people can never get enough of them!

Ten Tips to More Creative Energy

1. Be open to new ideas, less set in your ways.

2. Take time to daydream.

3. Gain a broad knowledge base, read more and read a variety of things.

4. Consider even the most far-out possibilities.

5. Deliberately create variety in your life. Break old patterns.

6. Ask "what if?"

7. Be spontaneous.

8. When you see something, ask how it can be done differently and better.

9. Go with your first hunch.

10. Try to be positive and optimistic.

11. Put ideas away, don't judge them, let them simmer. They'll come back better on their own at another time and place.

12. Think out loud.

13. Share a wild idea with someone else, bounce ideas off others.

14. Maintain a high activity level.

15. Remember, creative people never stop at ten!

Now let's switch gears and do a 180-degree turn from creative energy to logic energy. In other words, let's get logical.

7

LOGIC
ENERGY

Logic Energy

While creative energy is basically free-form and freewheeling, logic energy involves an objective, analytical approach to problems, decision-making, and planning.

When we think logically, we examine cause-and-effect relationships. We view events in sequence, relying on observations, measurements, and data.

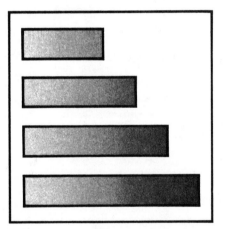

If you want to get more logic energy, you'll need to use the tools of the trade: a pencil or pen, paper (preferably graph or accounting), a calendar, and a calculator; and then prepare to put your life in order.

Why Do We Need Logic Energy?

Logical thinking seeks to understand cause-and-effect relationships by answering questions such as these:

- How did we get here?
- What are the next steps to take to get elsewhere?
- What will be the consequences of this action?
- Will this work?
- Why does (did) this happen?
- Does this make sense?

We need logic energy, in other words, to become more clear, concise, efficient, and effective. It helps us make the best use of what we already know; it helps us understand objectively which areas we need to know more about.

Perhaps the best-known example of pure logical thinking is *Star Trek's* Mr. Spock, who is always cool and analytical. His abilities, totally unclouded by emotion, have bailed The Enterprise out of many a nasty scrape.

Interacting With Other Energies

Logic is completely reliant on a sufficient amount of accurate, relevant information. Your prediction of outcomes can only be as good as the information it's based on. In computer jargon, this is called "garbage in, garbage out" (GIGO). We've already looked at how you go about collecting information from your senses or your intuition. But that information *must* be accurate.

None of us is Mr. Spock. As a Vulcan, he is void of emotions; we, fortunately, are not, but our emotions can go a long way to distort our logical thinking. We all have wishes, hopes, and fears, which are *subjective* emotions. Logic energy, remember, is *objective*, hence the conflict. Emotions can suddenly turn what should be an easy, clear-cut decision into a muddy, fuzzy, difficult one.

A special note to people with high-relationship energy: You probably won't "like" the suggestions in this chapter even though you may feel that they would be good for you. So here is a shortcut that a lot of our relationship-oriented friends have told us they use to deal with situations requiring logical decision-making: They talk to a highly logical friend who serves as a sounding board and helps them work through the pros and cons and come up with the best plan of action for the situation.

Logic energy involves four skills:

Skill 1: Problem-Solving. Including diagnosing, fact-finding, and decision-making.

Skill 2: Project Planning. Including goal setting, breaking down tasks into manageable steps, sequencing, scheduling, and project management.

Skill 3: Time Management. Involving setting goals, establishing priorities, and asking the question: "What is the best use of my energy right now?"

Skill 4: Predicting. Using model-building and formulas.

SKILL 1: PROBLEM-SOLVING

Is there a shortage of problems in your life? If so, you're abnormal. For most of us, problems simply come with the territory. Some of the problems in our own lives are major; they need immediate solutions. Others that are more minor can be put off (but that doesn't mean that they'll go away). And life confronts many of us with times when the accumulating problems seem endless or overwhelming, no matter how great our skills at solving them. Before we go on to examine problem-solving skills, though, let's affirm a point or two:

You're already an expert problem-solver. How do we know that? You wouldn't be able to face the problems of today as well as you do without having solved the problems of yesterday. You already have a solid, highly commendable history of successful problem-solving.

You can view problems as challenges. Being able to meet challenges has gotten you where you are today. You already know how to focus on a situation's opportunities instead of its obstacles, to turn a problem around and see how it can *serve* you rather than stop you. When you take your problems on as challenges, you remove many, if not all, of the emotional barriers that can otherwise stymie you.

Laying blame is no substitute for fixing a problem. You have to "own" a problem before you can solve it. And when you waste time and energy looking for scapegoats, you don't gain anything except some useless grudges. Get to work on a solution, not on finding culprits.

From the Bottom Up vs. Top Down

There are two approaches to problem-solving. The first uses what is called *deductive reasoning*. To solve a problem this way, you begin with an overriding principle and use that principle to establish a course of action for a specific situation. Guiding principles are well-established and often have excellent track records that will yield the right results when applied to different situations. A guiding principle in business, for instance, might be, "Minimize risks and maximize gain." In football, it might be, "Control the ball and you'll win the game." When you encounter a new situation, you reason from the overriding principle down— to quickly choose a course of action.

The second approach is called *inductive reasoning.* As the name suggests, this logic process starts with a specific situation and reasons up to the overriding principle or universal truth. When Sir Isaac Newton had an apple fall on his head, he asked, "Why?" Then he reasoned up to determine that gravity was the force that made the apple fall.

"A Thorough Diagnosis is 80% of the Solution"

That's a Chinese proverb, and while we can't confirm its math, there isn't any question as to its general wisdom. No matter which approach you take to solving a problem, your first step is to state it accurately. . .and in writing. How clearly can you articulate the problem and all its details? Answering these questions will help:

- What led you to conclude that there is, in fact, a problem?

- What's going on, as a result of this situation, that you find unsatisfactory?

- What do you have to gain or lose from solving the problem?

- What are your motives and underlying goals in addressing this problem in the first place?

In order to write a statement like this, you'll need to ask the right questions and find out where to get the right answers. By taking the time to define the problem this way, you're improving the likelihood that you'll make a good decision, and avoiding creating unnecessary additional problems.

Doing Your Homework

The scenarios below will help you see more clearly how to think problems through and approach your decision-making logically and thoroughly.

Let's say you're thinking about quitting your job and starting your own business, a not-uncommon conflict in everyday life. Too many would-be entrepreneurs make this decision on a snap basis—as a result of a fight with the boss, reading a single article that suggests the industry in question is about to take off, or an unexplained sudden burst of optimism. Unfortunately, all these are examples of emotion leaping in front of logic. There's a place in life, naturally, for some snap judgments, but the best long-term decisions are made by analytically asking and answering the appropriate questions. In this case:

- What kind of business are you thinking about? (Be as specific and detailed as you can.)

- Is there a market for your proposed product or service? How's it doing?

- Who are your customers/clients? Where are they? What kind of income/education do they have? How old are they? How many of them are there/will there be?

- How will you reach your customers, or have them reach you?

- Who presently serves your potential customers? How satisfactory is their product/service? What, if any, are the dissatisfactions with it?

- What will your start-up costs be (advertising, equipment, inventory, rent, etc.)? Be realistic; don't leave anything out.

- What will you live on for the next six to eight months? What resources are available to you?

- Whom do you need to hire? What personnel, with what skills? Where will you find them? How much will you need to pay them?

- What will make your business unique? Is this a "me-too" opportunity, or do you have a genuine competitive advantage?

- How can you use your present knowledge, skills, and experience to create sales for your new business?

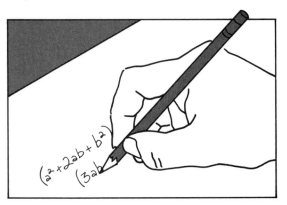

If you're indeed seriously considering the notion of your own business, by the way, *do not* skimp on any of these answers. Be as truthful and complete as you can. You're calculating your own future. Here's how you might go about finding the answers, if you don't already know them.

- Demographic studies. Demographics take into consideration statistical traits and characteristics (age, education, income, etc.) of a given population. A demographic study will fill in the blanks about your potential customers.

- Library research. Including periodicals, industry magazines, publications, and research via modem into computer data bases.

- Interviews with potential customers.

- Interviews with people who have enjoyed success in the field (and may or may not be competitors).

- Informed, objective people you can use as a "sounding board."

- Studies from government agencies and bureaus.

- Marketing firms. Even if you can't afford a full-scale analysis of your prospective field, often you can "pick their brains."

Even if the product or service you're thinking about is totally new and different, there ought to be something similar enough to it that the above questions and answers will be valid and relevant.

Logical Decision-Making: It's Really Simple Math

No matter how thorough or expert your information gathering, the problem you seek to solve will ultimately boil down to making a decision. One useful technique is to reduce the sides of the issue to a mathematical equation.

This process is sometimes called "Ben Franklin's Algebra," but it's really simple math. Its goal is to identify all the forces—both for and against—affecting your decision (including individuals, groups, fears, traditions, your expectations, and so on.) Some of these factors are readily apparent, some are not, and what Ben Franklin's Algebra accomplishes is to 1) incorporate all the information you've gathered and 2) identify and *quantify* all those positive and negative factors.

Let's apply Ben Franklin's Algebra to the same problem we began with: whether or not to quit your job and start your own business.

FORCES AGAINST	FORCES FOR
No certain income	Great income potential
Anxiety	Independence
Fear of failure	Get to be my own boss
Loss of fringe benefits	Challenge and personal growth
Insufficient savings	Can borrow the money
Can't see myself as boss	Have useful experience
Need new skills	Love this field; am capable of learning
Start-up costs	Initial investment soon recouped
Long hours	Flexible hours
Miss present co-workers	Won't feel trapped
Too difficult	Results worth extra effort
May not be fun at first	Will have more self-respect
Can't get my job back	Really need a change

Not all of the above forces will apply to you; you'd want to take three or four days to complete your own list. Your goal is to tease out all the factors that can and will affect your decision. You will want to talk to other knowledgeable people to see if there are additional forces you aren't aware of.

Now gauge the relative strength of each force by assigning a numerical value to it. (To introduce some objectivity into this process, it's often a good idea to have someone else look at the values you assign to these forces.) The scale is up to you, but the simpler you keep it, the easier your task will be; for instance, use a scale from 1 to 3. One represents a small force, 3 a very strong one. Let's look at it this way:

Transforming Stress into Power

1 = Has a slight influence on the decision

2 = Important; has moderate influence on the decision

3 = Very important; has a significant influence on
the decision

FORCES AGAINST		FORCES FOR	
No certain income	-3	Great income potential	+3
Anxiety	-3	Independence	+3
Fear of failure	-2	Get to be my own boss	+2
Loss of fringe benefits	-2	Challenge and personal growth	+2
Insufficient savings	-3	Can borrow the money	+3
Can't see myself as boss?	-1	Have useful experience	+3
Need new skills	-3	Love this field; am capable of learning	+2
Start-up costs	-3	Initial investment soon recouped	+2
Long hours	-1	Flexible hours	+1
Miss present co-workers	-1	Won't feel trapped	+1
Too difficult	-2	Results worth extra effort	+1
May not be fun at first	-1	Will have more self-respect	+1
Can't get my job back	-2	Really need change	+2
TOTAL	-27	**TOTAL**	+26

In this example, the forces "against" and the forces "for" came out about equal. (This won't always be the case; even with this example, different individuals might assign vastly different values to the same factors.) But regardless of the outcome, the next step is to examine the most important forces—your "threes"—and see if you can affect their impact.

FORCES FOR		FORCES AGAINST	
No certain income	-3	Great income potential	+3
Anxiety	-3	Independence	+3
Insufficient savings	-3	Can borrow the money	+3
Need new skills	-3	Love this field; am capable of learning	+3
Start-up costs	-3	Have useful experience	+3

This closer look shows us that the major obstacles to starting your own business are fear, uncertainty about money and income, and lack of knowledge about some aspects of running a business.

The first step to success is to minimize your risks before going on to optimizing your gains. So let's examine some new options (for instance, see the section on Brainstorming in the previous chapter), then apply our decision-making skills to those options. For example, you could take on a partner for your new business, sharing your risk. You could take a class or two in business accounting; write a business plan and use that plan to obtain venture capital or a small business loan; and so on. Those steps would ease your concerns about money/income and running a business; your newfound knowledge should alleviate your fear.

SKILL 2: PROJECT PLANNING

To plan a project, start with a known goal and a desired outcome. Successful project management increases your effectiveness and prevents you from wasting your time (or others') or having to redo things. It provides a measure to see how you're doing, and holds you and others accountable.

A successful project will usually have a definite beginning and end; it will require the coordinating and sequencing of people, resources, and activities. No matter how informal (planning a dinner party) or monumental (building a 55-story building) the task you're planning, the steps of project planning are the same.

1. **Establish your Goals**. Without goals, not only would there be no sporting events, but your entire existence would lack focus. Goals are challenges that serve to focus all of your activities; goals ought to be your main purpose. They are stressors in that they represent an

Transforming Stress into Power

ideal or future state that requires effort to attain, but that is a perfect example of how to put stress to positive work.

Write a goal statement of your project. This will tell you where you are going to end up.

2. **Chunk it Down**. Now break your goal down into measurable subgoals or "bite-sized chunks." Each chunk in this process is known as an objective; all objectives should be expressed in concrete, measurable terms so that you can tell when you've completed them. To "chunk down" is to work backward, beginning with the completed goal and ending with the present situation. For each chunk, develop a list of the major tasks to be completed and activities that must be performed.

3. **Organize the Parts**. Look at the project tasks and activities you developed in the chunking-down step. Now ask: "Which comes first? Which activities precede this one? Which activities follow?" Then put in order the tasks to be completed, taking into account the preconditions necessary for each step. For instance, a house builder would organize his project by foundation, flooring, walls before roof, electrical work, and finish carpentry.

4. **Estimate Resource Requirements**. It takes money, materials, people, know-how, and other resources to complete a project. Estimate the resources you will need for each project task. Develop a budget for each and for the total project.

5. **Sequence in Time**. Break down the total time you have to complete the project into smaller units. Now integrate the organized sequence of activities above into units of time. How long will activities take? How much extra time should you allow as a safe margin? How fast could you complete each step if you increased the person-hours, used another method, or used different materials?

6. **Create a Picture**. You might be able to put together a small project completely in your head, but to do larger projects, you will benefit from making them visual. When it comes to communicating something as involved and complex as a project, a picture is worth much more than a thousand words. Make a project flowchart, bar chart, or planning calendar. These can be used to monitor progress against your plan, to manage the total project.

7. **Celebrate**. The last step in any project is to celebrate. While not a true logic step, this last phase is important enough to reaffirm. With project planning you will be celebrating more successful projects completed on time, ahead of time, and under budget. Congratulations.

SKILL 3: TIME MANAGEMENT

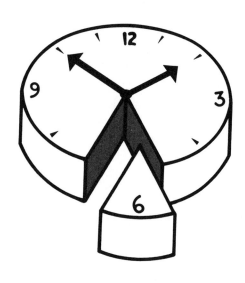

A day represents the same amount of time to all of us: 24 hours, 1440 minutes, 86400 seconds. Why, then, do some people seem to get so much more done in a day than others?

The answer lies in effective time management. Energy Directors structure their activities for maximum benefit. They use their time and direct their energy effectively to achieve both short-and long-term goals; they work smarter, thus get more done in less time.

One of the oldest of all business adages is: "Time is money." But in life, rarely do you get a thousand-dollar bill to spend all at once; similarly, you will not often have long stretches of uninterrupted time. Time management is more like investing "nickels, quarters, and dollars"— using short chunks of time more effectively. This ultimately adds up to "serious money" and major successes.

How do the Energy Directors do it?

● They write down their long-term goals (See Chapter 3, Direction), and make a daily "To Do" list.

● They use an organizer, such as an Executive Planner, Daytimer, or good desktop calendar. Whatever tool is actually used, the key is to have all your important information in one place, rather than scribbled on various scraps of paper or in your head.

● They establish priorities using the 80-20 rule. (80% of the value of what they do comes from doing 20% of the items on their list).

● They schedule higher priority activities so they can

tackle them when they're at their sharpest (for most people that means the morning, but you know yourself best). They save the lower priority activities, such as phoning, memo-writing, or filing, for a less productive time of the day.

- They hold themselves accountable for what they've done. This requires discipline as well as logic. They review their "To Do" list several times a day to check off what they've finished, and at the end of the day, they move unfinished items to the next day's "To Do" list.

- They avoid people who steal their quality or high-priority time.

- They ask: "What's the best use of my energy *right now*?" Then, they answer the question and they act.

One of the most valuable techniques to learn better time management is to keep a written time log for a week. Account for 15-minute segments of every hour. You may be surprised to find out where your time actually goes. Energy Directors become aware of how they spend their time and energy, make a decision to increase their effectiveness, and practice time management to get results. What is the best use of *your* energy, *right now*?

SKILL 4: PREDICTING: MODEL BUILDING AND FORMULAS

Ancient mariners who learned how to navigate with a sextant and determine their position on the open seas could sail far from the shoreline. With a sextant and some crude maps, it became possible to plan how to sail across the oceans and return. The power of models increased the range, freedom, and power of the captains who possessed them.

Today, models, which are abstract representations of the real world, are used by most of us whether we are engineers, scientists, designers, or business people. They give us the tools to make more informed choices. Models help us to understand how things work because they provide us with a way to visualize relationships between objects or thoughts; they help to structure our thought processes. They also provide us with a framework for understanding our experiences and a means of predicting what will happen next. We can use models to predict the effects of different courses of action to better achieve the outcomes we want.

Consider how you plan the route for a family motor vacation. Most of us get out a map and look at the highways we could take to get from our home to the vacation spot. We determine alternative routes, estimate the amount of time each would take, and choose a specific route. We are able to do all of this while sitting in the quiet of our own living room. Why? We have a model, the map, that has a one-to-one relationship with the actual roads and terrain we will be traveling.

Today's most complex models are mathematical. With the use of computers, engineers devise models and reduce them to the formulas necessary to place satellites into space. Models for human behavior, predicting the future of the economy or stock market, are far less precise. However, it is possible to develop models for these as well, or, for that matter, of anything.

You could create a model if you wanted to understand:

- how decisions are made in your company

- a customer's reaction to your marketing plan

- the best way to organize the furniture in your den

- how power gets from the engine to the tires of your car

- how cells reproduce

- how to landscape your home

With models, we can generate alternatives, test them in the model, and then choose the course of action that will give us the result we want.

The next time you are faced with a decision, take out a sheet of paper and develop a model. Or get out the computer and use a spreadsheet to answer "what if?" business questions. Models give you lots of power to test options and make great decisions.

Using these objective skills: problem solving, project planning, time management, and model building, Energy Directors increase their power in the real world. They reduce their distress by increasing their logic energy.

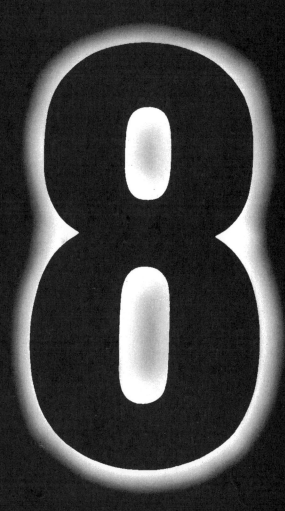

RELATIONSHIP
ENERGY

Relationship Energy

The Importance of Relationship Energy

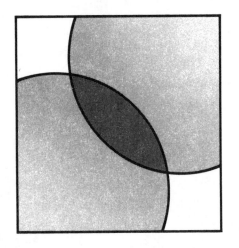

Relationship energy is the energy involved in feelings, emotions, values, intimacy, commitment, communication, friendship, and love. Not only do good relationships help us grow as people, but *they keep us healthy*—in fact, they help us live longer. There is considerable evidence that good solid relationships are just as important for good health and long life as exercise, nutrition, and preventive checkups.

Studies have shown that people with healthy relationships have less physical and mental illness than people who are socially isolated, and that close ties to family, friends, and community often result in reduced incidence of heart disease, stroke, circulatory diseases, and cancer.

Through relationships we learn to handle and re-direct stress more effectively. We develop greater self-esteem, which makes it far easier for us to hold others in esteem too. Relationships make us feel *connected* to life through others, and that's extremely important because the lives we lead often require us to work and interact with others to do things we just couldn't do alone.

If relationship energy is so essential to us all, the most important question is: "How can we get *more* of it?"

Emotional Sharing: The Core of Building Relationship Energy

To develop your relationship energy, you must look at *feelings* as a "unit of currency." And the way to build up "money" in your relationship bank account is through *emotional sharing*. All the tips, techniques, and exercises in this chapter are designed to help you relate emotionally to others. You'll also find additional information, specifically about long-term, intimate relationships in Chapter 10, Energy Directors at Home.

Building relationship energy is not an intellectual exercise, although people with high logic energy tend to approach it that way. In fact, you highly logical people reading this chapter may want to consider working on some of the suggested activities with a friend who is high in relationship energy. This person can help you by bringing a different perspective to the activities.

Getting Closer vs. Pushing Away

The first major step in building relationship energy is to understand that we all have the power either to move people in, or to push them away. Obviously neither move is all right or all wrong. People who are overly eager to move others into their lives may find themselves hurt by giving much more than they are getting. And people who go out of their way to push people away can become cold and reclusive.

Are you able to get closer to people when you'd like to or, on the other side, are you doing something that keeps significant others "at arm's length"? Let's examine how to keep your relationships in balance.

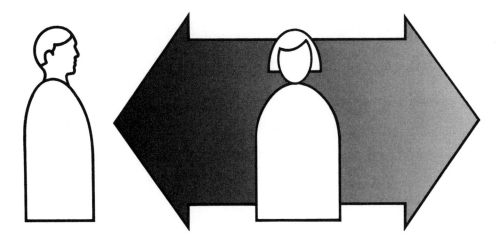

Here are some typical behaviors, some of which clearly act to improve relationships (getting closer), and others which result in building space into them (pushing away).

GETTING CLOSER	PUSHING AWAY
Listen	Ignore
Accept or observe	Judge
Share	Put yourself first
Open up	Close down
Ask questions	Remain aloof
Do something together	Avoid contact
Meet people at their level	Play "superior"
React positively, encourage	Discourage, discount
Smile	Deadpan or frown
Have a sense of humor	Be serious at all times
Show positive body language	Show negative body language
Maintain eye contact	Avoid eye contact
Praise	Criticize

Think about the current important relationships in your life, as well as one or two that, to your disappointment, have come and gone. How many of these behaviors can you recognize as yours? And can you see what your contribution to the relationship *really* was?

Naturally, our relationships with our spouses, parents, friends, colleagues, and bosses are not all the same. Relationships take on *levels,* and certain of those people will be more important or closer to us than others—more connected to our inner thoughts and feelings.

Transforming Stress into Power

It's normal for all of us to have relationships that have little depth to them—*brief contacts* such as the customers we see, people we talk to on the phone or pass on the street, people whom we chat with briefly as they serve us. It is not necessary for us to know all these peoples' names, and they don't need to know much about us.

Next we have *acquaintances*. We know their names; we greet them socially; we have some contact with them (perhaps to talk superficially about sports or the weather), but we don't express to them our inner thoughts and feelings. Many work relationships get to this level and stay there.

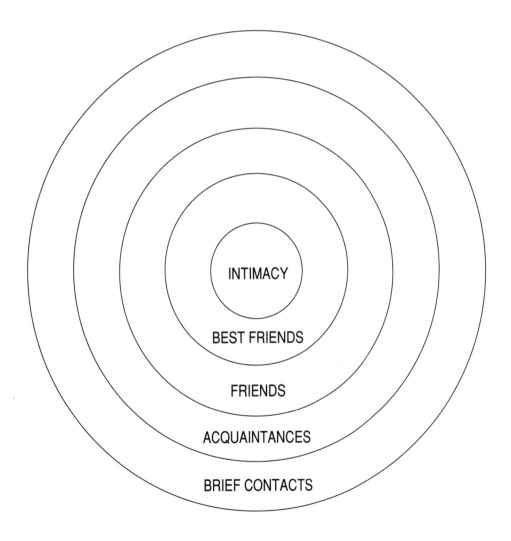

Our *friends* are on the third level. Our relationships with them escalate into our letting them get close to our real feelings and values. Almost everyone has his own definition of "friend," but let's say generally that a friend is someone who:

- has values and interests similar to yours
- you like to spend time with
- you share your important thoughts, opinions, and beliefs with
- you call upon when you're feeling down, and who will give you emotional support and encouragement
- cares about you.

And at the inner, core level, we have our long-term *best friends*. This takes in our lovers and, often, family members. We spend some of our highest "quality time" at this level, sharing our real vulnerabilities and innermost fears. With our best friends, we know that no matter what, we will still be valued, needed, appreciated, and loved.

At this inner core, many relationships take on the characteristics of *intimacy*—the loving quality of people sharing life's opportunities, mysteries, and challenges together. How do you know when it's right to be open and intimate, to make a long-term commitment to another? Here are some helpful questions to consider:

- Does this relationship bring out the best in me and in the other person?
- Does the other person make me feel more than what I am and can be by myself? Or less?
- Does this relationship make me feel good about myself and value myself?
- Does it help me move toward my goals and dreams in life?
- What is the effect of this relationship on me and on the other person?
- How do I really feel about sharing many years (the rest of my life) with this person?

Place the Names in Your Life

Here's an exercise that will help you identify the meaningful relationships in your life. Take a minute to make a brief list of the people you know who are significant to you. On the circle below, place their names according to the closeness of the relationship. How many people do you allow close, how many do you keep at "arm's length" (at a comfortable social distance), and how many do you keep permanently on the outside? Are there some people whom you'd like to move closer to you? Do you have a plan for doing it? Are there others who may be closer than you'd like, whom you need to push back a bit? To develop relationship energy, you'll want to move people closer by becoming more emotionally connected.

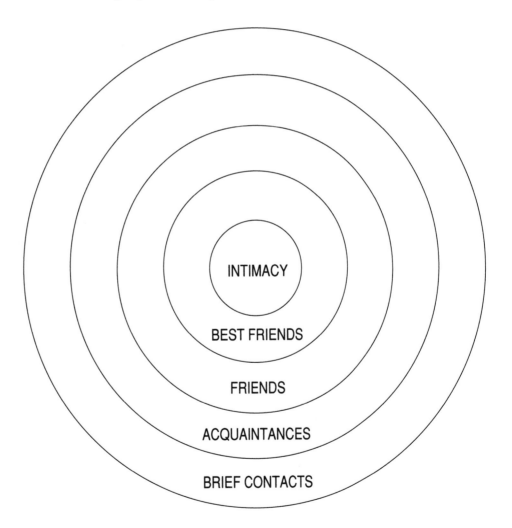

INTIMACY

BEST FRIENDS

FRIENDS

ACQUAINTANCES

BRIEF CONTACTS

An Easy First Step: Improve Your Listening Skills

One of the greatest stressors for high relationship people occurs when they feel that another person isn't really listening to them and attending to their feelings. To get more relationship energy, you must become a better listener.

Think for just a minute about how much time you spend listening each day and you'll quickly realize that it's one of the most important communication skills. But listening is a skill that many people have not mastered. Why? In part because it is all too easy to develop poor listening habits that continue throughout a lifetime. Scan the list below and see if you can identify your patterns.

1. *Lack of attention.* There's more to a message than just words. Listening demands a broad external focus: making eye contact, observing body language, conveying the impression that the other person's thoughts really matter to you.

2. *Frequent interrupting.* This tends to discount the importance of the other person's statement. How many times in a day do you interrupt someone in mid-sentence and not allow them to finish their thought? Several studies have shown that men do this more commonly than women.

3. *Listening superficially.* This is when you attend to the content but not the meaning. For example, a friend tells you about upcoming surgery. Instead of responding to his or her anxiety and concern, you ask a few shallow questions about the type of operation, the hospital, and the doctor.

4. *Rehearsing what you will say.* In this case you are so preoccupied with an internal focus (preparing what you will say as soon as there is an opportunity to respond) that you miss the entire content and meaning.

5. *Bracing for an attack.* In this case, you are expecting something negative, a hostile criticism or "scolding." Psychologically, you brace for the attack by shutting out any new input.

6. *Faking it.* Watch a politician in a crowd. The smile is there, the crinkle in the eye, the professional nod, but no real sincerity. When you act like a politician, the other person feels as though he or she is not getting through; you're a million miles away.

7. *Waiting for the expected.* Okay, you've heard this song and dance dozens of times; you know what's coming. You are so preoccupied waiting for it, that when and if the other person says something else, you totally miss it.

By correcting some of the mistakes above, you'll be in a better position to make more effective listening connections with others. But just what is it that you are listening for? There are three parts to the messages we receive from others. The first, and most obvious, is **content**. These are the facts: who, what, when, where—the basic information in the message. Most messages we receive each day stay at this level.

To develop your relationship energy, you'll need to listen for more than just the content of some messages—you must also listen for **feeling** and **meaning**.

When you listen for **feeling**, you try to receive the emotional impact of the person's message, the tone and texture that indicate how they have been affected by what they are relating. Body language, tone of voice, subtle behaviors are all clues to the feeling behind the message.

To listen for the **meaning** of the message, you must look for even deeper significance, somehow connecting the content and feeling with the person's deeper values and the ways in which he or she lives. Ask yourself, "What is the *real* meaning of what I have just heard?"

The Emotional Impact of Words

A good way to develop your ability to identify feelings and meaning is by examining the impact that words can have on others. People with high relationship energy often have a different vocabulary, especially of verbs, than others. Look over this list and try to sense the real feelings behind the word selection:

Adore	Share
Trust	Empathize
Feel	Care for
Cherish	Treasure
Love	Admire
Hurt	Grieve
Hate	

Are these verbs that you feel comfortable using when conveying feelings to others? Have there been times in your life when they might have been appropriate? If you didn't use them, what *did* you say? How did the other person react to your words?

If you are low in relationship energy, try using these (and other) relationship words more, noticing their effect on others; gradually you will develop a sense of the power of emotionally charged words.

Relating Emotionally

In order to relate emotionally to another, you must go beyond mere words and develop your own emotions to match the emotion being felt by that other person. Only then can you begin to act appropriately.

That matching of emotions is an area—really, an art—called *empathy*. Empathy is the willingness to place yourself in the other person's shoes and feel as he or she feels. It's not the same as sympathy, which deals only with feeling sorry for somebody; empathy carries with it connectedness and involvement. When you empathize with somebody, that person feels the sincerity of your response.

Think for a moment about a situation in which another person displayed a strong emotion such as anger, fear, or joy. Can you imagine what situation would make *you* feel as emotionally upset, distressed or elated? Now can you relate to their feelings?

Dealing With Feelings

Having feelings is an unavoidable part of being human. But feelings can be a major source of distress and tension, and dealing with them is a skill rarely taught in school.

Many people have been brought up believing that their emotions should always be held in check and be left unexpressed. If your parents always emphasized, "Don't cry; only babies cry," that's one common way in which that belief gets started. People who believe that their own emotions should be ignored or kept silent are frequently the same ones who ignore emotions in others. And both behaviors prevent the growth of relationship energy.

Expressing your own feelings effectively means you must refrain from trying to blame, judge, and heap guilt upon the other person; for example, "You made me do this. It's your fault." Such actions are usually met with the same sort of response: "Oh yeah, you're not so perfect yourself."

Begin by asking yourself, "How am I feeling as a result of this action?" Learn to express your feelings in the first person singular ("I feel...sad...mad...glad...angry," etc.). *Your* feelings are real and true for *you*. No one else can say they are wrong or can take them from you. Let others know how you feel by providing emotional feedback.

You'll also want to *ask* for emotional feedback, to know how something you did or said made the other person feel. You're going to have to accept that person's feelings as very real too. However inappropriate they may seem to you, they are true to that person, and you can't discount their being angry, hurt, or disappointed. Accept other people's feelings and emotions at face value.

How to Call a Cease-Fire

Accepting others' feelings and their point of view isn't always easy. Here's an exercise designed to help you take the other side.

Call a "cease-fire" (it's really more like a time-out), and each of you take a deep breath. Agree that for the next five minutes you will switch physical positions, and each of you will take the other's position in the argument. Be fair about it and argue your adversary's position with full emotion, conviction, and feeling; he or she should do the same with yours. At the end of those five minutes, stop and examine the points of agreement that have arisen (some should have) and build upon those points of agreement to resolve your differences.

The Beauty of Watching Relationship Energy Grow

One of the most rewarding sights on earth is watching the change in people as they develop relationship energy. They become gentler; they take on a new beauty; there is a sense of wholeness. This change doesn't occur in a vacuum; it occurs through commitment to others, through genuine caring, through an acceptance of life's joys and sorrows.

Ten Tips For More Relationship Energy

1. Celebrate your successes with others, celebrate others' successes.

2. Smile more.

3. Make contact with people. If appropriate, touch the other person.

4. Be available and give "the gift of quality time."

5. Do more for others.

6. Be more patient and accepting.

7. Try to see others' perspectives.

8. Appreciate and value yourself.

9. Anticipate another person's needs and do something special for him or her.

10. When dealing with others, don't just listen to what they're *saying*, try to hear what they're *feeling*.

Transforming Stress into Power

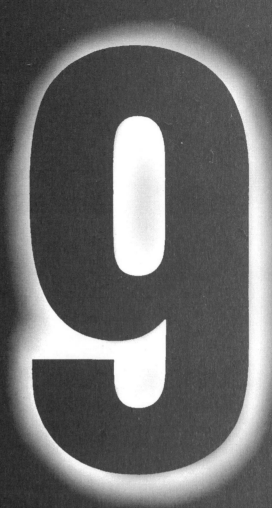

THE
ENERGY
DIRECTOR
AT WORK

Energy Directors
at Work

In our jobs, careers, and professions, we sometimes work as individuals and at other times we work as part of a team. In both cases, we have to know how to maximize our potential and be able to relate to our tasks and to the people we work with.

Just as there are healthy, high-energy people, there are also healthy, high-energy organizations. In this chapter, you'll find suggestions for maximizing your personal productivity, building high-energy teams, and healthier, more powerful organizations. We'll also provide a framework for the Energy Director principles and identify key questions to ask yourself and your team.

Personal Energy At Work: A Question of Fit

In earlier chapters, we've seen how important it is to be flexible—to be able to match the right kind of energy to the situation at hand. When selecting a job/profession/career, it is just as important that you choose one that builds upon your energy strengths.

Each person brings a different energy aptitude to the workplace; everyone is good at something. Efficient Energy Directors know how to adjust so that their skills meet the demands of the job. In the short term, they use the right kind of energy and direction for various tasks; in the long term, they choose a career that is a good match with their dominant energy.

Is there a best energy type for a particular job? The answer is, probably, "yes." Artistic jobs require high creative energy. Bookkeeping, accounting, and law tend to require high logic and high grounding energy, as does engineering. Health care and social service workers often have profiles that demonstrate high relationship energy.

Does this mean that one can't become a good accountant if he or she is a highly creative person, or won't succeed as a health care professional without high relationship energy? Absolutely not.

Although each of us has preferred energies, we can learn skills that will make us better-rounded people with increased career opportunities. It will be harder, and drain you a little more, to plan and develop a career on a weaker energy—at least until you've mastered the techniques. But it *can* be done.

It frequently happens that in the work setting we are "lured" into doing something—frequently for more money or a more stable future—that doesn't mesh well with our dominant energy. Again, this can work out if we can master the necessary skills—without undue distress during the process.

The Challenge of Focus

The vast majority of the mistakes that occur each day in the workplace are probably the result of a mismatch between energy (in terms of quantity, quality, and direction) with the demands of the task at hand. A much smaller number of mistakes are actually due to lack of competence—the absence of the specific skills to get the job done.

The same mismatches that cause mistakes on the job are also a major source of dissatisfaction with work, of boredom, and of burnout. Have you ever noticed how time flies when you are doing something you really enjoy? You're not looking at your watch, waiting for the minutes to pass. You don't feel tense, bored, or upset. That's because you've put all the right energies to work.

You can energize yourself each day by answering the self-examining questions on the next page.

1. Is this the best use of my energy right now? (That is, is it important or unimportant; and is it within my control or not?)

2. What type(s) of energy does this situation call for?

3. How should I direct my energy to get the best results?

4. How much energy will this task/job/problem/opportunity require, and over what period of time? (Do I need to gear up for a sprint or prepare for a marathon?)

Synergy and the Power of Groups

Now let's explore the nature of work relationships, and see how you can help teams work better.

Although it's a popular buzzword in business today (especially in mergers), the term "synergy" actually has its roots in pharmacy: two or more drugs or medications taken together increase each other's effectiveness (e.g. ergotamine and caffeine taken together to treat migraine headaches). Today, "synergy" basically means "the whole is greater than the sum of its parts." It's usually used to describe group power—how people working as a group can accomplish more than the same individuals working separately.

However you define synergy, remember that groups often produce more than individuals—and they may also produce results that are entirely unexpected. Those are two good points to keep in mind when you count on the synergy of a group to do a job.

Great Teamwork

Teamwork skills are the key to successful groups because teamwork is the key to synergy. You're part of a team; you have a "position" to play; others depend upon you to complete your work and you depend upon others so that the whole job gets done. This is synergy—the power of people working together.

Recall a time when you were part of a great group or team that got the job done well and felt good about it. Weren't most, if not all, of the following characteristics in that group effort?

Transforming Stress into Power

- *Good morale*
- *Cooperation rather than destructive competition*
- *The sharing of a common mission, goal, or vision*
- *A sense of being well meshed*
- *An emphasis on "we," not "I"*
- *Trust*
- *Open communication*
- *Give-and-take*
- *Support*
- *Follow-through on details*
- *Mutual respect*
- *Fun*
- *Celebration upon completion*

In short, a climate existed that allowed each person to feel appreciated. From the story below, we see that this feeling doesn't just happen by accident, it often must be consciously created.

Several years ago, we were brought in to work with the clinic staff of a large metropolitan hospital involved in conducting a research study on hypertension. The clinic had a problem with constant gripes, poor morale, and high turnover. The director asked us to investigate and determine if the clinic manager's style was causing the problem. We used a questionnaire and found, in fact, that the employees all held their manager in high regard. Another dynamic seemed to be the cause of the problems.

The most common feeling expressed by each member of the team was, "I'm the most important person here and I am not appreciated. I work the hardest; my job is the most important." Commonly these team members would compare themselves (how hard they worked and how good a job they did) to one or more of the other employees. The bottom line: no one expressed appreciation for each other's skills, talents, and contributions.

The group brainstormed ways to deal with the problem. The idea they came up with was to make certain to tell at least one person in the group one thing that they appreciated about them each day. Each team member checked off on the bulletin board that he or she had done so, and a healthy series of little "strokes" started emerging, like,"Jenny, I really appreciate the fact that you took care of Mr. Jones' test earlier;" "Thanks, Jim, for cleaning out the coffee pot, today...."or "Thanks, Gail, for rushing that through for me. It made a world of difference."

Energize yourself and your team with an appreciation for individual differences. While everyone goes about doing business in different ways, all have useful qualities that they bring to the job. Some are racehorses, some are turtles; some prefer planning projects, others prefer carrying them out. Learn to make allowances for approaches to problem solving that aren't necessarily your own.

Balancing the Energy on Your Team

If you manage a team, you have a unique challenge: assembling the right talent and then getting people with different talents to work effectively together. Here are some helpful questions to ask yourself:

1. Have we assembled people with the right energies to get the team's work done well? Are we:

- Getting enough data to make informed decisions (grounding)?

- Considering all the possibilities (creative)?

- Anticipating the consequences (logic)?

- Understanding how others will feel or respond (relationship)?

2. Are we providing a climate that appreciates and utilizes each person's unique contribution?

3. Is our team's energy focused to get the right result?

4. Are we celebrating and rewarding excellent individual and team performance?

Transforming Stress into Power

Of all the relationships we have on the job, probably the most important is the nature and quality of the relationship we have with our boss. It is not only a major determinant of job satisfaction and productivity, but also a major predictor of health. A poor manager-subordinate relationship can contribute to illness in the form of stress-related conditions such as ulcers, musculo-skeletal tension, headaches, etc. The goal for people who find themselves in such a situation is to get their boss "off their back" and on their side.

It takes time to build a solid relationship with your boss, one that will allow you to give your boss feedback on how his or her actions are affecting you. Sometimes it may be impossible, but it's certainly worth a try. You begin by doing two things: listening to and praising your boss. (In other words, the same treatment you would like to receive from him or her.)

By praise, we do not mean blanket flattery, i.e., "Gee, Mrs. Smith, every day I tell my wife what a wonderful boss you are and how happy I am to work for you." Praise, to be effective, has to be specific. It also must be sincere, and meaningful to the recipient according to his or her energy type.

For example, a woman attended one of our seminars and afterwards went directly to her boss to offer praise. She kept telling him how nice he looked—great tie, nice shirt—and found it wasn't working. The reason it didn't work is that she was appealing to his grounding energy (or lack of it). This boss was extremely high in creative energy. The type of praise he valued would concentrate on his new ideas, his vision, or his ability to see the "big picture."

Use the Right Type of Praise

People with high logic energy respond best to praise that acknowledges the soundness of their decision-making; people with high grounding energy respond to praise for their attention to detail, their follow-through, and getting the job done; and relationship-oriented people like to receive praise for their concern for others, their support, their ability to open lines of communication, and their handling of people.

Putting the Power of Energy Direction Into Sales

Imagine for just a moment that you could generate an Energy Director Profile on your prospective buyers. You'd learn their strong energies and the best ways of approaching them. You'd know whether to slant your pitch to emphasize the pros of your product/service and the cons of another (logic); to discuss the world of new possibilities that are available (creative); to highlight the sturdy durability of your product/service track record and its practicality (grounding); or to focus on the commitment you have to the product and the customer (relationship).

You could approach the sale from all sides if you had enough time, but one will be the best—particularly when it comes to closing the sale. Close with what is valid and true for the customer. Now you can't very well give the customer a quiz, but you can make an educated assessment.

First, listen to customers' questions and answers. What type of words do they use? Are they interested in ideas and concepts, or specific applications of the product or service? Watch how they approach the product. How much time do they spend touching and examining it, or trying it out?

Is your buyer concerned and sensitive to how others in the office might feel? Remember to note the tone of voice—relationship people classically have a softer, gentler tone, and will attend more to you. High-logic people are "crisp" in their tone. Chances are they'll want to review a cost/benefit analysis and more quickly get to the bottom line.

If you call on customers in their offices, look for pictures of and drawings by their kids (again, indicating relationship energy.) Look at the books in their office: are they scientific journals and technical publications, or books on innovation, teambuilding, and customer service?

You can easily blow the sale by not effectively handling your customer's major stressor. For grounding people, possible stressors include: not knowing how to use something, the fear of new technology, the thought that everything is changing, or uncertainty about the details of the deal. Creative people, on the other hand, will not fear changes or improvements; their concern will be for multiple uses of the product or service, possible product extensions, and its potential to grow with the company. Logic-oriented people are stressed by not knowing how a service or product will be received by the public, or by having doubts about its long-term profitability. And relationship-oriented people will be troubled by the lone nagging question of how happy their customers or office staff will be.

In addition to responding best to a specific type of praise, managers often have different expectations of performance that relate to their preferred styles. You must communicate with each different type based upon that person's energy, not yours. It's a matter of using the symbols, words, and approach that each type requires.

A manager in one of our seminars related a stressful, and enlightening, story...

There was a stressful time in my life when I was temporarily reporting to two bosses. They were as different as night and day. I'm high in creative and relationship energy. Boss #1 works the same way I do. I had some ideas for a new marketing plan, but I needed $50,000 to make it happen. I presented the concept and highlighted the possibilities to Boss #1. He responded, "Great idea. We'll look good. It will position us well with those customers. Okay, go talk to Dan." I left feeling really great, pumped up, and enthused.

I walked into Boss #2's office with the same pitch. After ten minutes, I got the feeling that he hadn't heard a word I said. In a nutshell, he let me know that I shouldn't waste his time without doing my homework first. I asked several people who had been reporting to him for their advice. They told me to submit a written proposal at least a week in advance, schedule an hour of his time, and be prepared to present a thorough analysis of the situation—including different options I'd considered and the process I went through to choose the recommended course of action. They also mentioned that I'd have a greater chance of success if I prepared a preliminary cost-benefit analysis.

The key to developing a relationship with your boss lies in knowing that person's energy preferences and being prepared to communicate using his or her language.

Building the High-Performance Organization

Organizations are teams of teams. For the purposes of this chapter, your team might consist of hundreds or thousands of employees, or just you and your spouse in the family business. The principles of energy direction are the same: to harness and direct individual and group energy to reach the organization's objectives, and to apply those energies to the organization as a whole. As a result, your organization has a personality of its own. But just as individuals get into trouble by overusing their dominant energy, so too do organizations.

Too Much Logic Energy

We've worked with a computer engineering firm whose high-logic energy engineers spent all their time improving the technological sophistication of the company's products. These engineers were happy working on formulas and theories in the isolation of their laboratory. Recently, their firm suffered serious declines in sales and profits because demand for the newly improved models was much less than anticipated.

Had the engineers spent more time listening to their customers, they would have learned that there was no demand for the new "bells and whistles." In this case, additional relationship energy would have kept sales volume up and customers happy.

Too Much Relationship Energy

Consider the social service agency helping run-away kids. The employees of the agency are all relationship oriented. Their training and education is in counseling and social work. Their manager is people oriented. He cares deeply for kids and is committed to doing everything possible to help them make it. This agency suffers from chronic staff burnout. Employees never say "no." Outreach activities bring in more kids to an already overloaded work force. Employees routinely work 10 to 12 hour days just to keep up.

What's the solution? More logic energy. The staff needs to put limits on its time. Schedules need to be made and priorities for helping kids must be established. The activities of the organization must be structured to increase effectiveness. Alternative methods for helping kids need to be evaluated. Staff members must learn to say "no." Burnout of agency employees can be reduced through planning, scheduling, and prioritizing.

Too Much Grounding Energy

We know many owners of small businesses who insist on doing all the work themselves. They enjoy tending to the landscaping, stocking the shelves, counting the receipts, writing the checks. Their customers leave satisfied, but their business does not grow. This is fine until a major change occurs that totally disrupts profitability, e.g. a dip in the economy, a technological improvement in the industry, or a new thrust in the marketplace.

Transforming Stress into Power

With more creative energy, small business owners could see the big picture, grasp trends in markets, discover ways to expand or modify their business to meet new demands. They would take some risks, learn some new ways of working and new skills for getting the business done. Successful entrepreneurs need to use large amounts of creative energy to make their businesses grow.

Too Much Creative Energy

They called themselves the "Jonathan Livingston Seagull Seven," a reference to the popular book about letting creativity soar. They were a small marketing firm that specialized in bringing a fresh approach to industries' problems. Hired by the company's founder, the key personnel mirrored his exact energy profile. With one exception—Ralph—they all showed high creative and high relationship energy. Ralph had a totally different profile: high-grounding, high-logic. During their brainstorming sessions, Ralph was frequently criticized for his inability to lighten up and let his imagination take flight. He wanted to slow down, take one step at a time, gather more data, and analyze the pros and cons before racing off and acting. Feeling unappreciated, he quit the company.

Several months after Ralph left, the company developed what it thought was a brilliant, far-reaching marketing campaign for its major client. The problem was, the campaign was so disjointed and impractical that no one could understand it. The "Six" lost their major account. A little more grounding energy in the person of Ralph (or someone like him) could have resulted in a more focused, practical approach, and better relations with the client.

Natural Biases

These stories demonstrate the need to balance the energies within an organization and, in larger companies, to resolve the natural conflict between different departments. Manufacturing is really biased toward grounding energy; Sales is generally composed of relationship-oriented people concerned with keeping customers happy; Research and Development (R & D) personnel are known for their creativity; and Finance relates everything to the "bottom line." Businesses present normal conflicts because different energy types dominate the different departments. Research and Development may run up against Marketing, Sales against Manufacturing, and so on. Obviously each function, and its supporting energy, is valuable and needed, and each must be blended into the whole.

To determine an organization's personality (and often its financial health as well) our customary method is to ask four questions, each relating to specific energies. This helps us to see corporate "distortions" when one kind of energy goes out of balance. Consider:

1. Does your organization regularly collect and use information from your markets, competition, and the external environment?

2. Do you have ongoing processes that promote creativity, innovation, and risk-taking for product and service improvements?

3. Do you have structures and systems to effectively use information for decision-making and utilize resources for productivity?

4. Do your people *feel* that they are the organization's most valued resource? Do your customers *feel* that you value, listen to, and care for them?

If you answered "no" to any of the above, be prepared to provide the missing energies needed to balance out the company's total energy profile. For example, firms that are "too soft" (have too much relationship and creative energy) need strategy, structure, accountability, measurement and data collection. Firms that are "too hard" (too much grounding and logic energy) can achieve balance through team building, rewards and recognition, a people-oriented culture, and more face-to-face contact with their customers.

Transforming Stress into Power

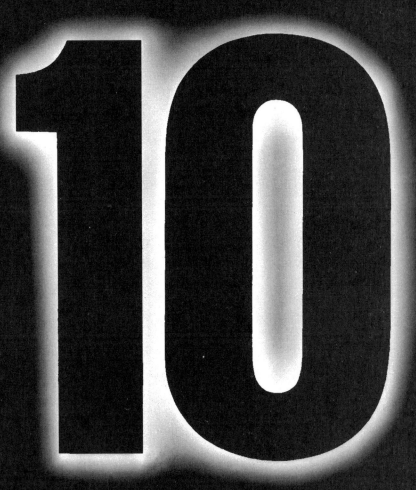

THE ENERGY DIRECTOR AT HOME

10

Energy Directors at Home

Now that we've had a closer look at relationships with friends and co-workers, let's examine the closest relationships of all in your life. What's going on at home?

A satisfying home life is obviously heavily dependent on good relationship skills. The way you apply your relationship energy at home could actually be called "family energy." The primary source of this kind of family energy is the quality and dynamics of the relationship between you and your "significant other," whether or not you are married to each other.

This chapter looks at family relationships from an energy perspective. We'll discuss how to rekindle the sparks of your loving relationships, how family communications can get fouled up, how to help your children develop their unique energies, and how to help them balance out their weak points. We'll examine the family as a team and build some strategies for creating a happier, healthy family unit.

The Dynamics of Bonding: A Parable

Once there was a beautiful willow tree that grew near a strong, sturdy oak. The willow admired the firmness with which the oak stood against the wind; the oak appreciated the willow's soft, yielding nature, and its ability to bend and sway with the same wind. The two became attracted to each other. They grew closer and closer so that their roots began to intertwine.

One day the oak said to the willow, "Why don't you stand up a little straighter? You should be more like me, stronger, tougher, not moved so easily by every wind."

"Oh, the problem with you is you're so rigid," replied the gentle willow. "You think your way is the only way. You're so stiff, you think everybody should be just like you and the world would be fine. It wouldn't hurt you to learn to bend with the wind a little."

After years of criticizing each other's different qualities—the same qualities that attracted them in the first place—the two decided they could not live together. Neither was willing to allow the other to grow the way it wanted. So they moved apart, separated their leaves and branches, and tore the one-root-ball structure apart.

They divorced, and each tree went into shock.

Do you truly love another person just the way that person is, or are you in love with a fantasy that you are trying to make that other person fit into?

The warmest, longest-lasting relationships are almost always those in which the couple accepts—without judging—one another's uniqueness. The commitment they make to one another is one of freedom and growth, but the cement that holds the whole thing together is their *bonding*—their growing together while allowing each other to grow separately too.

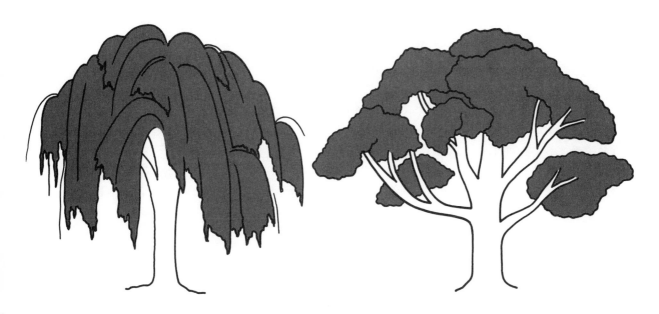

Appreciating the Differences, Reinforcing the Similarities

If you haven't already done so, we encourage you to have your significant other complete the Energy Profile in Chapter 3. Compare his or her profile with your own. In what areas are you unlike? Are there any similarities—strong energies that you share in common? There are three different patterns that we commonly see in couples.

In the first pattern, individuals become attracted to and fall in love with a mate whose energy is the exact opposite of their own—someone who has qualities that they themselves lack. A cool, analytical, ordered, structured, logical person becomes attracted to a warm, emotional, high-feeling, relationship-oriented person. A person with high levels of freewheeling, blue-sky creative energy bonds with a grounded person who exists in the here and now, is practical and sensation-oriented, and focuses on getting results.

When we see another person's ability to complement us in that way, it makes us feel "complete" or "whole." There are few finer feelings in this universe—yet there's still the possibility that what was once attractive can become a constant irritation (as in the case of the fable of the oak and willow). If one party has an energy preference for constant logic and the other for empathy and concern for feelings, the two may come to measure and contrast their preferences instead of continuing to harmonize.

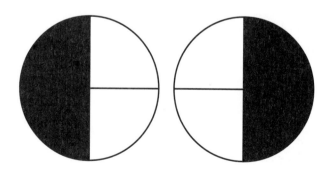

The second pattern is seen in couples having one of the energies strongly in common. This at least, even though they differ in the others, gives a base to the relationship— a sense of familiarity that perhaps makes it easier to share experiences and relate to the other person.

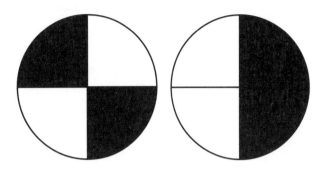

The third pattern occurs when two people have the exact same profile. We believe this can lead to high quality relationships when the two people each have a high level of self-esteem and feel confident about and comfortable with their own energy profile. When this comfort level does not exist, fireworks can ensue. We saw this recently in a marriage between two high-logic people, both of whom were attorneys for large law firms. They were so much alike that they engaged in logical one-upsmanship; each tried to out-analyze the other.

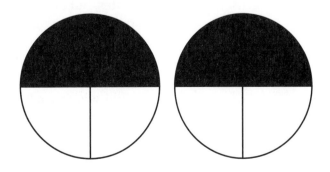

Putting the Spark Back in Your Love Life

At one point, your significant other was the center of your universe, the passion of your life. But time and circumstance dull this feeling. How can you put the spark back in your love life?

To begin the process, you start by accepting that person just the way he or she is. You can't change other people, can't mold them into what you want them to be. Their energy profiles were cast long before you met them.

The key is to constantly recall that, at one point, you saw in your mate some unique energies that you valued and appreciated, and you let the other person know it. Whatever you did in the courtship that won the affection of your mate must continue throughout the relationship.

It's the little things that begin to count. Write a love letter to your mate. Set aside special, high-quality time. Have a secret ritual that you share. Use the affectionate name you used when courting. Leave work early and take that person on a date. Reaffirm the one you love by expressing admiration and respect. Make it clear that you want to continue living your life together.

Remember, the bond you have with your mate is the core of family life, and for better or worse, it will be mirrored in all your family relationships.

The Family Magnet Game

As you probably know from science class or from magnetic toys, two magnets of opposite charges will attract each other, and two of the same charge will repel one another. And, of course, you recognize by now that some human relationships can behave the same way.

This is true not only of the relationships we form with our mates, but also of those we form with our children. All parents would like to be fair and treat each of their children equally as to love and caring; many may think they do. But in reality, that's an ideal that rarely takes place. No matter how hard we try, there is usually one child whom we like better. We get along better with that child, and he or she becomes our "favorite."

At the same time, we may find that we "dislike" the traits of another child by comparison, so that child becomes a target of constant criticism. We insist on comparing him or her to the favored brother or sister and trying to correct and/or change aspects of the child's behavior. No matter what that kid does, it rubs us the wrong way.

The best way to keep those conflicts from becoming more pronounced is to understand our own energy preferences—and understand how our children are developing their own energy skills. Not only can you help your kids develop their strong energies, but you can help them balance their weaker ones as well.

Understanding Your Child's Energy Profile

Does your child have the same energy profile as yours? If so, you as a parent may be very critical of that child, and try to help him or her avoid the same mistakes you made. If you're creative, you may find it difficult to praise, value, and develop that same creativity in your kid. You probably criticize that child's lack of being grounded too; parents are always after their kids to put things away, to stop daydreaming, to do practical things, to pay attention to the real world.

Accordingly, be warned that parents can sometimes be too hard on kids. If you're not comfortable with your own energy patterns, you may become very critical when you see those same patterns in your children. Be certain not to take out your frustrations on them.

Some parents may have just the opposite tendency: they are most critical of the child or children with the energy type exactly opposite their own, especially if it mirrors the profile of their spouse. The result is that their relationship with that child often parallels some of the dynamics between husband and wife.

By recognizing your and your mate's energy profile, you'll be better able to appreciate the individual differences that make people unique. And, as you'll see from the next section, you'll be better able to identify your kids' dominant modes of acting.

The Nintendo Preference Story

Shortly after Christmas, our wives went shopping with Steve's three children— Celine, age 8, Jesse, age 7, and 6-year-old Ryan—to purchase another video game for their new Nintendo system. All the way home the kids debated the new game from their own clearly defined energy-preference points of view.

Ryan: "Let's look at the box first so we'll know how to play. If we don't and we do the wrong things, something will kill the spaceship."

Jesse: "No Ryan, let's just figure it out as we go along. I don't care if my spaceship dies. You can play this game forever. And we might figure out some ways to play that aren't even in the rules."

Celine: "Let's just all have fun and play it together, but don't fight about it."

Each child's approach to the Nintendo game, to school work, and to life in general, mirrors the child's energy preference. Ryan's strong suit is logic energy. He likes order; he wants to go by the rules and not make any mistakes.

Jesse sees possibilities and options in all that he does. He is high in creative energy; in this case he's looking for ways to play the game that may take him well beyond the boundaries of the written instructions.

Celine is our Social Directress. For her, the fun of being together and playing together is far more important than winning or losing, or the creative possibilities, or the rules.

Children from age one to five seem to be into grounding energy. They taste, touch, manipulate, explore, and delight in discovering the sensory world. They live totally in the present. Later, from age six to 12, they start developing strong relationship, logic, and creative energies. In children this age, energy preferences are already highly developed.

So how can you help your child? There are two ways. The first is to steer your children toward activities and careers that will take advantage of their strong energy. For example, in the story above, Ryan shows early tendencies that could help him excel as an attorney. Jesse might do well as a research and development engineer. Celine already wants to be a teacher or a camp counselor. The key is not to lock in and limit your children's future career choices, but to guide them into careers where they have a natural advantage for doing well.

The second step parents can take is to help children develop their weaker energies.

To Build Creative Energy

Let your kids fantasize. Ask them to look at clouds and describe the animals and other things they see in them. Let them describe imaginary friends they play with. Let them know it's okay for them to make up stories and pretend. Encourage them to tell you about their dreams and listen to them. (Even "scary" dreams are a form of inner creativity.) Read stories together; encourage your children to describe their vision of the characters.

Play the games they like to play, but change the rules and create unusual approaches. Encourage them to draw make-believe pictures. Let them know that you think creating is both fun and valuable. Years later your children will remember and appreciate you for helping them develop their creativity.

To Build Logic Energy

Let your kids work out projects. Ask them how they think things happen. For instance, have them describe what will happen if you drop something, move something, start a ball rolling down the driveway. When they ask, "Why?" give them reasons. Don't say, "Because I said so, " or "Just because." If you don't know the answer, say "Let's go find out."

If they want to know, for example, why glass, which is made out of sand, is clear, get out an encyclopedia and read together about making glass. Go to the library and look up the story of glass making. Help your children develop the habit of asking logical questions and seeking answers and solutions. Encourage them to think things out and figure out answers to problems. Show them how to use numbers and formulas to figure out simple things. Ask them to help you measure distances and estimate the amount of materials needed to do some weekend projects.

To Build Relationship Energy

Encourage your children to explore and express their feelings. When conflicts develop, help them get in touch with and "own" their emotions, rather than blame someone else for how they feel. Let your kids know that you value and appreciate tenderness. Tell them how good their hugs and kisses make *you* feel.

Give each child the gift of your undivided and full attention. For example, make certain to spend a few minutes with each child before bedtime. Ask if there is anything the child would like to tell you; inquire about what happened that day. This quiet time together often provides an opportunity for sharing hurt feelings and personal joys. Remember to model the loving feelings you want your child to have. The easiest way is by sharing feelings of tenderness and concern with your spouse.

To Build Grounding Energy

Nature has most likely already seen to it that your kids are curious, love to explore things, and have good healthy levels of grounding energy. Don't squelch those natural inclinations. Encourage them to use that energy to explore and experience their world. Offer them opportunities to make things with their hands; give them help if it's needed. When you drive somewhere with your kids, play "The License Plate Game" (who can spot the most states and the most letters of the alphabet). When you take your kids for a walk, ask them to identify colors, sounds, and smells. In this way you *guide* children toward the magical discovery of their sensory world.

Sports are another great learning forum where kids can develop their grounding energy (provided you avoid today's terrible over-emphasis on *winning*). Participation in sports not only helps kids refine their grounding energy, but it builds sensory motor skills, competence, and confidence. In athletics, the mind and body are coordinated into a single purpose, therefore both are grounded masterfully.

Will all your kids become fully balanced Energy Directors? Probably not. But over time, you can help them become more rounded and better able to live fuller, more successful lives. By learning to understand their unique patterns, you will also be able to relate more effectively to them during times of stress.

My Mom is the World's Greatest Worrier

You might be a worrying mom, or you might have one, or both. In either case, when you're a mother—or dealing with one—worry is part of the job description. And no matter how much love passes between mother and children, mothers are very capable of making their children and themselves half crazy with worry.

Hovering, over-protective mothers are an example of relationship and creative energy running amok. Their seemingly endless nit-picking and meddling usually comes from love; indeed, one of the things you hear most often from others about such mothers is, "She means well."

There isn't any question that a mother's concerns are very, very real. It's her *expression* of these concerns that causes problems. The concerned mother is not aware of her actual impact on others; she is so busy expressing her concern that she can't see the effect of her message. And, at the other end of the communication, we don't receive her message clearly because it seems all cluttered up by concern, guilt, judgment, and a sense of urgency. The following is a typical example of such a mixed message.

"Did you see the article in *Parade* magazine about all the kids who hurt their heads when they fall off their bikes? Don't you ever let my grandchildren ride in the street without a helmet. It's dangerous. They could break their necks. God forbid that my grandchildren could become statistics. And you know how wild Billy is, he doesn't pay attention to *anyone*. I can't believe you're letting him ride in the streets that way. You go out and get a helmet right now!"

The message is one of genuine concern, caring, and love for the grandchildren—but while we say something like, "Okay, mom, whatever you say, "our real response is likely to be along the unspoken lines of, "Get off my back."

Less often, we might respond more honestly, but in an adversarial way: "Look, you always tried to tell me how to run my life, now you're doing the same thing with my kid. My kid can do whatever he wants. He's mine, not yours."

A better solution for everyone would be to look for the **meaning** of the worry, and attend to that meaning. "Gee, mom, you're really concerned about this, aren't you? You're right; it is important. Thanks for calling it to my attention. I've seen grown-up motorcyclists wearing helmets, but I never thought about it for the kids. I want Billy to be as safe as possible, too. I'll ask our doctor about it."

Or you might have a great mom who shows up one day on her bicycle, wearing her helmet, and delivering helmets for all her grandchildren to use. No advice given. None needed.

Helping Your Kids Deal With Stress

Bob Henley was promoted from Plant Manager to Sr. Vice President of Human Resources, a substantial jump up the corporate ladder. In the career sense, this was a good positive stressor for Bob. His wife supported the move, but when he announced it to his three kids, he saw only distress.

The move meant a disruption of their family life, leaving Cleveland, their home for the last eight years, and moving to Connecticut. The three kids were accustomed to the city—the two youngest had never lived anywhere else—and the entire family was happy with Cleveland as a place to live and grow.

Each of the three children responded differently. Bob, the oldest at 12, and Jenny, the youngest at seven, became angry and initially responded with denial and anger. "We don't believe it...you can't do this to us." A few days later, Bob was able to sit with them, logically go over the pros and cons, and help each of them analyze the decision, and see its benefits in a new light.

But for Tim, the middle child, it was a different story. At age eight, he didn't ventilate his feelings at first as the others did. When they were expressing their anger, he kept telling them, "It'll be okay. Don't worry. We'll make new friends there." Tim, naturally high in relationship energy, sought to comfort his brother and sister. He took it upon himself to be the emotional "glue" that carried his siblings through the crisis.

Yet, a few weeks later, Tim burst into tears in his mother's arms sobbing, "I'm sooooo scared..." He had attended to the needs of the family, showing his concern for harmony and everybody else's feelings—but, unlike his brother and sister, he didn't get a logical explanation of the move because no one realized he needed help.

The solution was for Bob to make some special, or "quality," time for Tim, and share his feelings. He expressed vulnerability ("You know, it's hard for me, too; I'm probably more nervous than you are.") He showed appreciation for Tim's helping and caring for the others. This is Energy Direction at its best: Bob related to Tim using the energy that was real and valid for Tim.

All parents have the tendency to rescue their children, to want to solve all their problems for them as opposed to letting them work them out. But after doing your best to help your kids grow more competent, there's a point at which you simply have to let go.

Families: Working Together, Working It Out

The healthiest family relationships all involve working together—working out problems and taking advantage of opportunities. You'll enjoy even more happiness in your home when you learn to direct your energies toward recognizing each person in that home individually— your mate as well as your kids. Spend "quality time" with your entire family, and learn to appreciate what makes each member special. If you do, you'll be more likely to have a family that's together emotionally for life.

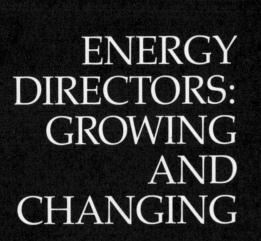

ENERGY DIRECTORS: GROWING AND CHANGING

Energy Directors: Growing and Changing

Tom and Jenny: Not Enough in Common

Let's revisit the four people we met in Chapter 3 and see how they are working out their energy patterns and relationships.

Tom (high logic energy: cool, analytical, and objective) and Jenny (high relationship energy: warm, caring, and sensitive) were at first very attracted to each other. There were times when they really seemed close, in fact, a natural fit. But after a year of serious dating, what started out feeling "so right" became more and more of a struggle.

Jenny was at first attracted to Tom's calm, objective reasoning. She viewed his ordered life as a stabilizing force—the exact opposite of her highly emotional life filled with friends whom she needed and who needed her. But in time, Jenny came to resent what she saw as his coldness, unwillingness to open up, lack of commitment, and his inability to share feelings. He just didn't appreciate her emotions and was not sensitive to her needs and moods. Worst of all, he didn't do enough of the "little things" that made her feel special, desired, and happy.

To Tom, Jenny was a loving, caring, supportive woman who made him feel good. He basked in the love and nurturing she gave so completely. Her warmth and personal attention were a welcome contrast to his world of objective analysis and impartial decisions. But, as time went on, it seemed he was in a battle with her. He began to feel uncomfortable with her strong feelings and the way in which she made decisions; he felt she resented his objective approach. She wanted him to warm up and spend more time with mutual friends. Tom began to perceive her "caring" as an "intrusion" and to view her "concern" as an attempt to change him into something he wasn't. He thought he would never be able to meet her emotional needs and demands. Eventually they broke up.

Tom Connects with Others

Several years later, after a lonely period in his life, Tom came to realize that he had become a workaholic who had failed to develop his personal life. He started reading about relationships and attended a human growth seminar. He began to get in touch with his emotions by listening more closely to others and attempting to respond to their feelings as well as the content of conversations. He started to realize how much he had been missing. Slowly, he came to appreciate some of the traits of high-relationship people and to be more comfortable with them.

Tom started slowing down and gradually became more aware of his own emotions. He made an effort to see situations as others see them. As Tom warmed up, friends opened up more to him, too, and shared more about their lives, hopes, pains, and dreams. Ultimately he was able to commit to a relationship with a very special woman. Tom still tackles life's challenges first with logic, but he is increasingly aware of the feelings of others.

Jenny Gets It All Together

Jenny married a few years later. She works with her husband operating a rapidly growing retail computer business. The company sells hardware and software and provides custom-designed installations for many businesses. As her life became more and more complex— she had two children, fourteen months apart—it required greater planning. Jenny started making "to do" lists, establishing priorities, and creating action plans. By doing so, she found herself becoming better able to handle the demands placed on her.

Jenny learned to use a computer to operate the business and became comfortable working with spreadsheets to project its growth. While she appreciates the power and logic of the computer, she feels most comfortable dealing with customers, anticipating and meeting their needs. With her high relationship energy in sales and her growing use of logic and computers for operating the business, Jenny is building a successful operation. She still tends to emotionally overextend herself, but has become better at using logic to set priorities. She will frequently do a pro- and con- analysis when faced with a major problem, or talk things out with a high-logic energy friend.

Logic energy helped Jenny solve one of the stressors she endured for years: worrying unnecessarily about other people. She doesn't play the "worst case worry game" any more. ("What if something bad happens to one of the children or my husband?") When tempted to do so, she sits down and examines the likelihood of something happening (very slight) and the amount of energy she is expending on needless worry (enormous). Gradually, Jenny has learned to put many of her fears aside. She has begun to focus more on the important things that she can control, and to worry much less about things that are either unimportant or uncontrollable.

Two Friends Who Helped Each Other Grow

Now let's revisit Charlie and Barbara, members of the art museum fund-raising committee—they've become friends. Barbara (high grounding energy: "be here now," woman of action) convinced Charlie (high creative energy: an idea a minute, new ideas and possibilities) to take up racquetball. At first it was really difficult for him. Then he began to find something very satisfying about the simple activity of hitting a ball and directing it where someone else couldn't hit it. As Charlie started playing four or five times a week, he found that the physical activity gave focus to his blue-sky existence. Gradually, he began to follow through on projects to their completion, pay greater attention to detail, and to act more effectively on his creative ideas. His staff now notices that he is able to focus more clearly on their problems, where in the past he brushed them off. With Barbara's help, Charlie has learned to build his creative ideas upon a solid base of sensory information.

Charlie encouraged Barbara to keep an idea journal, to doodle more, to let go of some of her set ways of doing things, and to look at situations in a totally new way. He shared with her one of his brainstorming techniques: how he begins each project by looking up the key word or concept in a thesaurus, then allows his imagination to develop images based upon the different words.

With Charlie's encouragement, Barbara tried applying some of her newfound creative energy to her work at the bank, specifically with some of the bank's client companies. She found creative visualization helpful, for example, to "see" how some of these companies would grow in the future. Barbara still feels most comfortable with the "real" world of facts, figures, and hard evidence, yet she is starting to use creative energy to anticipate and prepare for the future challenges facing her financial institution.

As Barbara's skills have broadened, her superiors have begun to consult her about new services for the changing needs of the bank's customers. (By the way, Barbara and Charlie worked out a great fund-raising campaign for the art museum that included many innovative financial and creative programs. For example, one allowed people to donate property to the museum in exchange for a life-long annuity. This generated a large endowment for the museum and provided long-term security for the donor.)

It *Is* Possible to Change

In the examples above, the four individuals have not magically developed their weakest energies and solved all of their problems overnight. Each continues to primarily use his or her strongest energy, but they have also learned to make that extra effort to develop their weakest energy and use it appropriately. By doing so, each person has gained valuable skills for meeting life's demands and capitalizing on opportunities. They have also come to better appreciate people whose dominant energy is different than their own. They demonstrate flexibility and a willingness to change and grow; they are learning to transform stress into power. You can do the same. Now it's up to you.

Your Personal Action Plan

In Chapter 1, we outlined a six-part technique for change, beginning with awareness and ending with mastery. Ten chapters later, let's review these steps.

1. Awareness

What insights and realizations have you gained by reading *Transforming Stress Into Power*? What have you found out about yourself? How comfortable are you with what you have found? Have you become aware of some predictable patterns that get you into trouble? How do these relate to your dominant energy? Most important, do you have the desire to change? Are you willing to make a commitment to become your best? If not now, when?

2. Knowledge

By now, you've gained a better understanding of the dynamics of stress, and why desires and demands require energy. But you also know that you need to not only match these stressors with the right *amount* of energy, but also to use the right *kind* of energy and to direct it appropriately. You've determined your unique Energy Profile and, hopefully, the profile of some people who are important to you. You've identified your dominant energy and your weakest energy. And you've gained an appreciation of individual differences.

3. Techniques

Take a moment to look over the chapter that deals with your weakest energy. Can you see some advantages to improving in that area? Choose one or two of the techniques in that chapter for getting more of that energy and reread those sections a few times. Consciously choose to attend to those techniques and develop your Achilles' heel. You might want to review the tips and techniques for your strongest energy as well, and refine it even more.

4. Practice, Practice, Practice

In reality, this is grounding energy in practice. Reading about change, thinking about it, imagining the possibilities, is a start, but there's no substitute for action. Start *using* your techniques. At first, you may feel a bit awkward or self-conscious. That's normal; don't give up. You might see if you can find a "coach" to help you develop that energy.

5. Skills

These come through practice over time. You know you have a skill when you use the technique that best meets the energy demands of the situation...and you get the results you want. As your skills develop, so too does your personal power, the ability to be effective and in control of your destiny.

6. Mastery

Perhaps the best definition of mastery is "doing the difficult with ease." Those who have mastered a sport, an art form, or the skills of a profession make it look so easy. They have achieved a level of competence and confidence that allows them to just be themselves. The years of building awareness, acquiring knowledge, practicing techniques, and developing skills have culminated in a remarkable and unique set of abilities.

In our work, our travels, and our lives, we have met some masters. These are the people who have served as our role models.

They live their lives with heightened sensitivity and awareness. They are able to use their energies effortlessly. They add just the right blend of creativity to some situations to make the impossible possible. They bring logical objectivity to situations that are confusing and chaotic. They give the gift of quality time and respond with emotional warmth and sincerity. They act at the right time to get the right result. These masters of energy direction can be found in many places. Take the time to find them. Watch them. Use them as role models, and have fun celebrating the energies of life.

The Energy Director Party

Want an idea for a party game that's more fun than Trivial Pursuit, more entertaining than Pictionary, and a lot more meaningful than Monopoly? Try our recipe for an Energy Director Party. It's ideal for a group of from 12 to 40 people. Here's all you need to play.

THE INGREDIENTS

- One copy of the Energy Director Quiz (page 15) and Energy Director Profile (pages 41-45) for each participant. (You can photocopy these from this book.)

- Ten or 12 large pieces of butcher paper, newsprint, or chart pack pages (two feet by three feet or larger)

- Masking tape

- Five or six colorful, large-tip marking pens

THE GAME PLAN

Step 1: Introduce the concept of the party: namely, that each person will learn more about his or her strong and weak energies.

Step 2: Have each person fill out the Quiz and Profile.

Step 3: Divide guests into groups that are named after the four energies. (Make sure you have at least two people for each energy. If not, borrow someone who's fairly strong in that energy from another group.) Keep groups together in same room to receive further instructions.

Step 4: Provide each group with several sheets of paper and a marker. Have the groups elect a "recorder" who will write down the group's answers. (If you decide to have groups attach the paper to the wall with masking tape, make sure the ink doesn't "bleed" through onto the wall.) Remind the recorder to write the group's energy type at the top of each page.

Step 5: State the following, "Your group is composed of experts on your particular energy. Please take the next thirty or forty minutes to carry out the following five tasks I am going to give you and to record your answers. When all the groups are finished, we'll get together and make presentations." Now send each group into a different room (or a different corner) and give each group a copy of the following instructions.

THE INSTRUCTIONS

1. What tips, hints, and techniques do you recommend for people low in your energy to gain more of your energy? (In other words, if you are in the high logic group, what could other people, not high in logic energy, do to be more like you?)

2. List your main stressors.

3. What is a good motto or saying to describe your energy?

4. Draw a symbol or a mascot for your energy.

5. Finally, create a skit, draw a poster, or develop an advertisement you can present to others to convince them that *your* energy is the most important of all.

Step 6: After the groups have finished, bring everyone back into the large room and ask for volunteers to present their work. Encourage each group to act out its skits or advertisements. Let people ask questions, make catcalls, and generally give the other groups a lot of feedback.

You'll be amazed at how quickly people playing this game start to appreciate each other's energies. If they want to know more about energy direction, tell them to read our book.

We hope that holding an Energy Director Party will be fun for you and your friends. It will be an evening of entertainment and, just possibly, the beginning of a lifetime of insights.

Transforming Stress into Power

About the Authors

Mark J. Tager, M.D.

Mark Tager is President of Great Performance Inc., a Portland, Oregon, based consulting firm that specializes in health promotion, management development and culture change products and programs.

Dr. Tager received his medical degree from Duke University and trained in Family Practice at the University of Oregon Health Sciences Center. A dynamic keynote speaker and trainer, he has conducted programs and retreats for clients such as Northern Telecom Inc., AT&T, IBM, Procter & Gamble, James River Corporation, Bristol-Myers, Merck Sharp and Dohme, Exxon, The Internal Revenue Service, The American Association of Homes for the Aging, The Prudential Insurance Company of America, John Alden Life Insurance Company, Blue Cross Blue Shield of Illinois, and Tektronix.

Dr. Tager has served as Director of Health Promotion for the Kaiser Permanente Medical Care Program in Portland, Oregon. He organized in-house prevention programs, designed organizational strategies, created marketing programs, established health policies, and trained personnel in leadership skills.

Dr. Tager has been actively developing communications for the public since 1975. He has written several books including *Working Well: Managing for Health & High Performance* (with Marjorie Blanchard, Ph.D., Simon & Schuster, 1985); and produced more than two dozen educational films.

Stephen E. Willard, M.S.

Steve is an energetic trainer and consultant who has presented seminars to thousands of business and government leaders in the United States and Asia for over fifteen years. His vitality and enthusiasm are contagious. Participants return to their workplace and make changes that increase productivity, creativity, team and personal performance.

Steve is owner of a small business and knows the reality of building companies. As a consultant to many businesses, he has helped them to increase sales and profits, and to sell internationally. His clients include multi-national corporations such as Phillips, Intel, and San Miguel Corporation. He has extensive experience in county and state government, both as a manager and as a consultant.

He has a B.A. degree from Whitman College and a M.S. degree from Portland State University.

YOUR UNIQUE ENERGY PROFILE

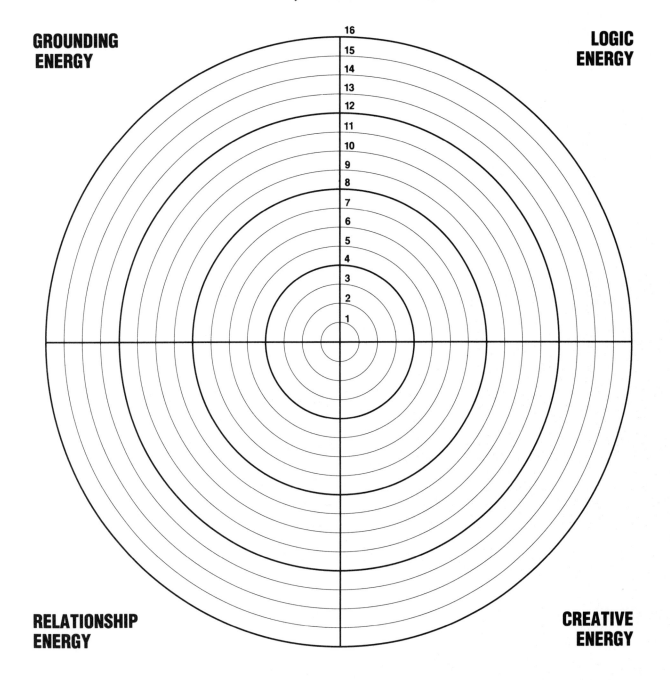

YOUR UNIQUE ENERGY PROFILE

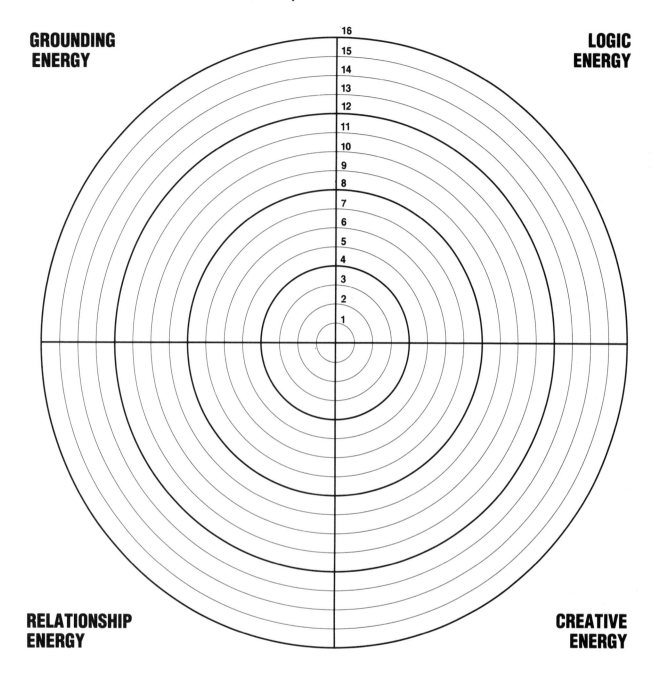

GROUNDING
ENERGY

LOGIC
ENERGY

RELATIONSHIP
ENERGY

CREATIVE
ENERGY

16
15
14
13
12
11
10
9
8
7
6
5
4
3
2
1

ORDER FORM
1-800-433-3803

☐ YES! I would like to order, at no risk*, the following Great Performance materials at the prices shown, plus shipping and handling.

TO: **GREAT PERFORMANCE INC.**
14964 NW Greenbrier Parkway
Beaverton, OR 97006

☐ YES! I would like to receive free of charge the Great Performance catalog.

SUBTOTAL _____

Quantity	Great Performance books, audiotapes and videos	Code	Price	Amount
_____	*Transforming Stress Into Power,* book and 4-audiotape set by Mark J. Tager, M.D. and Stephen Willard	EDA1	$39.95	_____
_____	*Transforming Stress Into Power,* 30-minute video by Mark J. Tager, M.D. and Stephen Willard	EDVU	$95.00	_____
_____	*Personal Action Sampler*: sixteen 16-page, 4-color health and wellness guides. Topics: *Stress Management, Cholesterol Control, High Blood Pressure, Nutrition, Fitness, Back Strength, Women & Self-Care, Alcohol &Drugs, Walking,Weight Management, Healthy Relationships, Wellness, Smoking, AIDS, Diabetes* and *Men &Self-Care.*	PK209	$32.95	_____
_____	*Designing Effective Health Promotion Programs: The 20 Skills for Success Workbook* (128 pp. spiral bound) by Richard Bellingham, Ed.D. and Mark J. Tager, M.D.	WB103	$19.50	_____
_____	*Working Well: Managing for Health and High Performance* (240 pp. hard bound book) by Marjorie Blanchard, Ph.D. and Mark J.Tager, M.D.	B101	$15.95	_____
_____	*Working Well* audiotape by Mark J. Tager, M.D. and Marjorie Blanchard, Ph.D.	AV101	$9.95	_____

Ship to: _____
PLEASE
PRINT   _____
_____
_____
_____
_____

Sales Tax or Exempt #_____
(Add applicable sales tax for
IL, OH, MI, IN, WI, TN)

Shipping / Handling _____
Add 7% (minimum $5.00)
Allow 2 weeks for delivery.

TOTAL ENCLOSED _____

METHOD OF PAYMENT

☐ Charge to AMERICAN EXPRESS
☐ Charge to VISA
☐ Charge to MASTERCARD
☐ Check enclosed

Card Expires_____ /_____
Card Number_____
Signature_____

*If for any reason you are not completely satisfied, the materials can be returned with 15 days for a full refund.